Cardiac Rhythm Disturbances

Disturbances

A STEP-BY-STEP APPROACH

Cardiac Rhythm Disturbances

A STEP-BY-STEP APPROACH

WILLIAM FOX, M.D., F.A.C.C.
  Clinical Assistant Professor, Department of Medicine, The University of Chicago
  Director of Cardiology, MacNeal Memorial Hospital, Berwyn, Illinois
  Diplomate, American Board of Internal Medicine and Subspecialty Board of
    Cardiovascular Disease

EMANUEL STEIN, M.D., M.P.H.
  F.A.C.P., F.A.C.C., F.C.C.P.
  Professor of Medicine and Professor of Community Medicine, Eastern Virginia
    Medical School, Norfolk, Virginia
  Formerly, Medical Director, United States Public Health Service
  Diplomate, American Board of Internal Medicine and Subspecialty Board of
    Cardiovascular Disease

Lea & Febiger • *Philadelphia 1983*

Lea & Febiger
600 Washington Square
Philadelphia, Pa 19106
U.S.A.

Library of Congress Cataloging in Publication Data

Fox, William,
  Cardiac rhythm disturbances.

  Bibliography: p.
  Includes index.
    1. Arrhythmia—Diagnosis. 2. Electrocardio-
graphy.   I. Stein, Emanuel,
II. Title. [DNLM: 1. Arrhythmia—Diagnosis.
2. Electrocardiography. WG 330 F6655c]
RC685.A65F66   1983   616.1'2807547   82-12727
ISBN 0-8121-0838-8

PRINTED IN THE UNITED STATES OF AMERICA

Print No.   5   4   3   2   1

In loving memory

GITEL ROTHMAN

(1886–1965)

Our Grandmother and Aunt

PREFACE

This book was written to enable individuals possessing elementary knowledge of electrocardiography to become proficient in the interpretation of cardiac arrhythmias. It is designed to be of use to medical personnel ranging from CCU nurses to practicing cardiologists. Indeed, it is the authors' firm conviction that the art and science of electrocardiographic interpretation does not depend on an M.D. degree or on a certain level of clinical proficiency. However, the book does assume mastery of basic skills and concepts, such as what are P-waves and QRS-complexes; determination of QRS axis; identification of right and left bundle branch block patterns.

There are four Sections, each encompassing major groups of arrhythmias. Each begins with a text that discusses the various arrhythmias, with emphasis on electrocardiographic characteristics and variations, differentiation from other arrhythmias, and the methods of analysis and their pitfalls. In addition, electrophysiologic and clinical background is provided where appropriate. The electrocardiograms (ECGs) then follow. Their order of appearance roughly parallels the discussion in the text; in addition, within each group of arrhythmias, the ECGs progress from the simple to the more complex. Individuals who are more advanced may quickly review the early, straight-forward ECGs, and go on to dwell on those presenting more difficulty or complexity. For all but the simplest ECGs, the interpretation provided includes a step-by-step analysis, so that the reader may learn how the conclusion was reached. Indeed, the goal of the book is not only to present a compendium of arrhythmias, but also to teach an analytic approach that can become incorporated into the thought processes of the reader. Those completing the book may continue to use it as an encyclopedia, to refer both to examples of the various arrhythmias, as well as to interpretations encompassing certain trains of thought or methods of analysis.

The designation of every Table, Figure, and ECG contained in the book is prefixed by a Roman numeral indicating the Section to which it belongs. Thus, Table I-1 and ECG I-48 are both located in Section I. Upon completion of the book, the Tables, Figures and Electrocardiograms can be rapidly located for reference and review.

This work is an outgrowth of the material presented for a number of years in electrocardiography teaching conferences. Participants are asked to interpret arrhythmias projected on a screen, and, in cases of difficulty, are guided through the analysis, step-by-step. It is in this spirit that this book is written.

Chicago, Illinois   William Fox
Norfolk, Virginia   Emanuel Stein

CONTENTS

SECTION I

Supraventricular Rhythms and A–V Dissociation

INTRODUCTION

In this section, the characteristics of normal sinus rhythm as well as the various supraventricular arrhythmias and forms of A–V dissociation will be discussed. All involve QRS-complexes produced by electrical impulses arising above the bifurcation of the His bundle (hence, the term "supraventricular"). These QRS-complexes are usually narrow (0.06 to 0.09 sec.) and have a normal morphology, unless altered by bundle branch block, myocardial infarction, ventricular hypertrophy, or other disturbances.

Normal Sinus Rhythm

The S–A node is located high in the right atrium, near the entrance of the superior vena cava. The cells of the S–A node are endowed with the property of *automaticity;* that is, they have an electrical diastolic drift toward threshold, which, when reached, results in an electrical discharge. The S–A node, or "sinus," is normally the fastest of the heart's many centers of automaticity; it is therefore usually the dominant pacemaker of the heart.

Normal *sinus rhythm* (SR) arises in the S–A node. The electrical impulse thus formed normally spreads *via* specialized internodal tracts to the A–V node, thence the bundle of His, bundle branches, and terminal Purkinje network before activating the ventricular myocardium. Activation of the atrial myocardium from the sinus node produces a "sinus-P-wave," having a mean electrical frontal plane axis of −10° to +90° (in most cases between +15° and +75°). Sinus-P-waves are flat to upright in Lead I, upright in Lead II, and usually upright in aVF; the Lead II contour is either monophasic or somewhat notched. In the horizontal plane they are upright or biphasic (positive-negative) in Lead V_1, and although frequently of low amplitude, upright in Lead V_6. Following a P–R interval of 0.12* to 0.20 sec.,** the sinus-P-wave is followed by a supraventricular (narrow) QRS. To diagnose SR, one must see a rhythm consisting of such sinus-P-waves, each followed by an appropriate and constant P–R interval and QRS, with a P-wave preceding each QRS, and a QRS following each P-wave. The usual rate is 60 to 100 beats per minute (bpm). SR whose rate is above this range is called *sinus tachycardia; sinus bradycardia* if below this range. Because of the changing autonomic influence on the S–A node accompanying respiration, there is usually a slight phasic variation in the heart rate. When this variation exceeds about 10%, *sinus arrhythmia* is said to be present. In most cases, a normal degree of variation is preserved even at rapid heart rates, and this fact may help differentiate marked sinus tachycardia, in which such variation is usually present, from *ectopic atrial tachycardia* (PAT), in which it is usually absent.

In some cases of SR, the P–R interval may be prolonged (up to 0.60 sec.). This usually bespeaks

---

*In occasional cases, the P–R interval is less than 0.12 sec. This may be caused by a heightened adrenergic state, or by an A–V bypass tract ("Lown-Ganong-Levine syndrome" if narrow QRS; "Wolff-Parkinson-White syndrome" if QRS has initial slurring ["delta wave"]).
**Maximum of 0.21 sec. below rate of 60 bpm.

A–V nodal delay, and is called *first degree* (1°) *A–V block*. Given a greatly prolonged P–R interval and/or faster heart rate, the sinus-P-wave may occur in the T-wave of the preceding beat or, in marked cases, preceding the antecedent QRS itself. Vagal maneuvers, (Table I–1), such as carotid massage, Valsalva, or edrophonium (Tensilon) administration, may, by causing a slight, transient slowing of the rate, separate the P-wave from the preceding QRS-T, enabling the correct diagnosis to be made. Sinus tachycardia is slowed by digitalis only when the underlying cause is heart failure.

Premature Atrial Beats (PAC)

PACs are beats originating from an ectopic atrial focus. They are characterized by early non-sinus-P-waves, occurring before the expected sinus-P-wave. The morphology of the PAC P-wave is usually quite different from that of the sinus; however, multiple leads may be necessary to distinguish between the two. Occasionally the difference is quite subtle ("peri-sinal" PACs, presumably originating close to the sinus node). Unless the rare condition of S–A node entrance block is present, a PAC always enters the S–A node and resets the sinus by one cycle-length. The interval between the ectopic P-wave and the subsequent sinus-P-wave usually equals one sinus cycle plus about 0.10 to 0.20 sec. During this additional increment, the PAC is in the process of reaching, entering, and discharging the sinus. In cases of a "sick sinus" (idiopathic or drug-induced), a PAC may depress the

sinus, so that the post-PAC beat is considerably delayed.

PACs are usually able to conduct to the ventricles, thus producing a QRS-complex which follows the ectopic P-wave by an appropriate P–R interval. Relatively late PACs, that is, those only slightly premature, may conduct with a normal (0.12 to 0.20 sec.) or even short P–R interval, the latter signifying an atrial origin relatively close to the A–V node. Earlier PACs, encountering a conducting system still partially refractory from the previous sinus beat, may conduct with 1° A–V block; the earlier the PAC, the greater the delay. As a rough "rule of thumb," a P-wave occurring beyond the T-wave of the preceding beat is usually able to conduct. Early PACs are occasionally timed so that the impulse, though able to traverse the A–V node, becomes blocked in one or more of the still-refractory bundle branch fascicles. The resulting QRS-complex is said to have *functional aberration* of the corresponding bundle branch (right bundle branch block, RBBB; left bundle branch block, LBBB, RBBB plus a hemiblock, or a hemiblock alone). The mechanism of functional aberration will be further discussed in Section III. Still earlier PACs find the conducting system completely refractory, and fail to produce QRS-complexes *(nonconducted PAC)*. When one sees an early QRS-complex interrupting an otherwise regular sinus rhythm, one looks closely for a premature P-wave in order to identify or exclude the beat as a PAC. The premature P-wave is often located in the T-wave of the preceding complex; here, one sees

TABLE I–1. Vagal Maneuvers.

Maneuver	Comments
1. Carotid massage	a. Contraindicated if bruit present; massage of carotid ipsilateral to side of hemiplegia contraindicated. b. Effect is potentiated by other vagal maneuvers and digitalis. c. If good effect is seen, potential benefit of digitalis is implied.
2. Valsalva	Contraindicated in acute myocardial infarction.
3. Tensilon (edrophonium)	a. Contraindications: allergy, wheezing after previous administration, significant bronchospasm. Relative contraindications: history of asthma, COPD, major GI disturbances. b. Administration: After test dose of 1 mg, give 5–10 mg IV. If maintenance therapy is desired, begin drip of 0.5–2.0 mg/min.
4. Pressor agents (e.g., methoxamine [Vasoxyl])	a. Action: produce vagal discharge *via* hypertensive effect on carotid sinus. b. Contraindications: hypertension; acute myocardial infarction or unstable angina (unless frankly hypotensive because of tachyarrhythmia). c. Indications: Reentrant supraventricular tachycardia with blood pressure low normal or frankly hypotensive, when the arrhythmia is unresponsive to other vagal maneuvers. d. Administration: begin IV drip (10–20 mg in 500 ml) and administer until systolic BP 160–180 mm Hg achieved (*do not go higher*). e. Note: Vomiting often accompanies breaking of the arrhythmia. *Blood pressure must be monitored minute to minute.*

deformity of the T-wave compared to one not containing the P. Occasionally, the PACs occur in *bigeminy*, that is, following each sinus beat; in this case, all the sinus-T-waves are deformed. Deformed T-waves are usually pointy, indented, or notched, compared to the smooth, round contour of the pure T-wave. During sinus rhythm, when an unexpected pause of the sinus occurs, one should always closely examine the preceding T-wave for deformity; a blocked PAC is often found. In fact, even where the rate is regular and uninterrupted, sinus-T-waves should always be routinely inspected for deformity. "Sinus bradycardia" occasionally turns out to be SR with blocked PACs in bigeminy. "Normal SR" occasionally turns out to be digitalis-toxic "PAT with 2:1 block" (to be discussed later).

Occasionally one encounters a bigeminal rhythm in which two apparent sinus beats are followed by a pause of greater than one and less than two sinus cycle-lengths. If the bigeminal pattern is precisely repetitive (i.e., all short and long cycles are equal), the diagnosis lies between SR with perisinal PACs in bigeminy *vs.* SR with 3:2 S–A Wenckebach periods (to be discussed in Section II). Examination of all 12 leads for minor differences in P-wave morphology must be undertaken, and, in the case of peri-sinal PACs, this will be found. If the bigeminal rhythm is not precisely repetitive, the differential diagnosis, in addition to the above two entities, may also include simple sinus arrhythmia with phasic cycle variation occurring in a pseudobigeminal pattern. Again, one would look for (1) subtle differences in P-wave morphology (suggesting peri-sinal PACs), and (2) changes in heart rate producing inconsistent S–A Wenckebach periods of the same ratio (i.e., the pattern and length of the

R–R intervals for all 3:2, 4:3, 5:4 periods, respectively, should be identical), or producing inconsistent calculations of the true sinus rate with different S–A Wenckebach ratios*—in either case, the inconsistency excludes S–A Wenckebach periods (see ECG II–49C).

Premature Junctional Beats (PJC)

Sometimes, a premature supraventricular QRS-complex is not preceded by a premature P-wave. One is dealing with a *premature junctional beat* (PJC), arising in the His bundle or the lower ("N–H") region of the A–V node (both areas comprise the "A–V junction"). The PJC preempts the normally occurring sinus-P-wave; that is, it may occur in the ECG so that it *precedes* the P-wave (early PJC), occurs at the same time as the P-wave, or follows it by a shorter than normal P–R interval (late PJC). If the heart rate is slow, a relatively late PJC may occur before the sinus-P-wave and be able to conduct back to the atrium, producing a *retrograde-P-wave*. Retrograde-P-waves are inverted in Leads II, III, and aVF, flat or upright in Lead I, and usually small, monophasic and upright in Lead V_1 (see Figure I–1). It is essential to remember that the actual PJC is the discharge from a His bundle pacemaker, and is not visible on the surface ECG. The supraventricular QRS-complex one calls a "PJC" is actually the ventricular activation resulting from the antegrade conduction of the true PJC. Depending on the relative speeds of ante-

---

*Suppose there are two beats and a pause, then three beats and a pause, suggesting 3:2 and 4:3 S–A Wenckebach periods, respectively. The sinus rate calculated from the 3:2 period should be the same as that calculated from the 4:3 period, if the clusters of beats truly represent S–A Wenckebach periods.

TYPICAL MORPHOLOGY

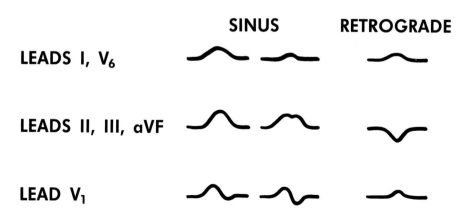

Figure I–1. Sinus- and retrograde-P-waves.

grade and retrograde conduction, the retrograde-P, when present, may precede, coincide with, or follow the QRS of the PJC. (When the retrograde-P precedes the QRS-complex, it does so by a P–R interval of 0.12 sec. or less, since *the retrograde-P does not produce the QRS, but, rather, both are almost simultaneously produced by the PJC.*)

If a retrograde-P-wave occurs, the sinus is reset by one cycle length (plus the usual 0.10 to 0.20 sec. for the retrograde-P to enter the sinus and reset it). If a retrograde-P does not occur, and the PJC precedes the normally occurring sinus-P-wave, that P-wave may or may not conduct to the ventricles, depending on the refractoriness of the conducting system following the PJC. Again, as a "rule of thumb," if the sinus-P occurs after the T-wave of the PJC, it usually is able to conduct. If it falls earlier, it may conduct, but with 1° A–V block; earlier still, and it is unable to conduct (in which case a "full compensatory pause" occurs—that is, the interval between the conducted sinus beats surrounding the PJC is equal to two sinus cycle-lengths).

PJCs, like PACs, are subject to the various degrees of *functional aberration.* This fact is of importance, because it is possible for a PJC producing no retrograde-P-wave to encounter *complete (trifascicular) functional block* in its antegrade conduction, thus, also producing no QRS; should the next sinus-P-wave follow this "concealed PJC" in short order, it may find the local junctional area still refractory from the PJC, and also fail to produce a QRS. Since the PJC without its antegrade or retrograde products (QRS and P, respectively) is invisible on the surface ECG, the above situation appears as a *sudden dropped beat* ("pseudo-Mobitz II block," which will be discussed in Section II).

Premature beats may also arise in the proximal bundle branch fascicles.* Although, strictly speaking, not supraventricular in origin, these *premature subjunctional beats* (PSJC) are closely akin to PJCs. It is often not possible to differentiate between PJCs with functional aberration and PSJCs. One must find a *very late* premature beat; if it still has a BBB pattern, it is likely to be a PSJC.

Finally, the electrophysiologic mechanism for the production of PJCs and PSJCs is unclear. Unlike most PACs, which probably result from a discharge of an ectopic focus of automaticity, PJCs and PSJCs may actually result from a mini-reentry circuit in the His bundle or bundle branches. This

mechanism is postulated in part because, while PACs may occur in salvoes, PJCs and PSJCs occur only singly. It is known from clinical electrophysiologic studies that only single His/bundle branch reentry beats can be produced. Of course, PACs, PJCs, or PSJCs which are not coupled to the preceding sinus beat by a constant interval (i.e., are not "fixed-coupled") may actually represent atrial, junctional, or subjunctional *parasystole,* respectively. (The mechanism, namely, a latent focus of automaticity which acquires protection from the dominant pacemaker, will be discussed in Section IV.)

Ectopic Atrial Rhythm

These rhythms arise from an ectopic atrial focus which has become, usually transiently, the dominant pacemaker. An ectopic P-wave precedes each QRS, usually by a normal P–R interval. If the ectopic focus is located in the low atrium close to the A–V node, the P–R interval may be short (0.08 to 0.12 sec.). The P-waves differ from sinus-P morphology by being biphasic, notched, inverted, etc., in various leads. "Coronary sinus" rhythm (inverted Ps in II, III, and aVF) and "left atrial" rhythm (inverted Ps in I and V_6; "dart and dome" P in V_1) are merely two of the many patterns of ectopic-P-wave morphology seen. When the ectopic P-waves look like classic retrograde-Ps (negative in II, III, aVF; flat or upright in I; monophasic and upright in V_1) and the P–R interval is short (0.12 sec. or less), differentiation between ectopic "low" atrial rhythm and *"high" junctional rhythm* may be difficult,* but when the patient is young and in good health (the usual setting for these rhythms), this differentiation becomes academic. Ectopic atrial rhythm occurs at rates generally ranging from 40 to 100 bpm, with most at 50 to 75 bpm. Occasionally an ectopic atrial focus may control the heart for long periods of time and vary its rate according to autonomic influences (e.g., accelerate during exercise, etc.). However, at some point, usually at faster rates, the sinus resumes as the dominant pacemaker. When the rhythm changes from ectopic atrial to sinus, and *vice versa,* the new rhythm may first appear as either a premature (early) beat or an escape (late) beat. In some cases, the atrial morphology may gradually shift between the two ("wandering pacemaker"). As with sinus rhythm, ectopic atrial rhythm may be

---

*The QRS morphology exhibits the appropriate patterns of BBB—e.g., RBBB + left anterior hemiblock, if arising from the posterior fascicle of the left bundle.

---

*In some cases the differentiation can be made. For example, a change in the P-wave morphology or resumption of the sinus at a slower rate suggests ectopic atrial rhythm; constant R–R intervals with retrograde-P-waves finally disappearing into the QRS implies junctional rhythm.

interrupted by PACs. Finally, a focus producing *paroxysmal (ectopic) atrial tachycardia* (PAT, to be discussed later) may occasionally also appear as one or more beats of ectopic atrial rhythm after the PAT terminates.

Wandering Atrial Pacemaker

This is basically an ectopic atrial rhythm in which the site of the atrial focus varies. Some sinus beats may also be present. There are at least three separate P-wave morphologies as well as some variation in the P–P and P–R intervals.

Salvoes of PACs

Two or three or more consecutive PACs may occur in close order, producing a heart rate of 100 to 250 during the salvo. The PACs may have constant or varying P-wave morphology.* If more than 6 to 8 beats occur, one is said to be dealing with a short run of PAT (constant morphology) or *multifocal atrial tachycardia* (varying morphology). Since the salvo begins with a PAC, the first and possibly subsequent beats may show functional aberration.

The Supraventricular Tachyarrhythmias

A mechanistic classification of the various supraventricular tachyarrhythmias is given in Table I–2. *Sinus tachycardia,* which has already been discussed, results from some underlying clinical problem (fever, hypoxia, heart failure, hyperthyroidism, etc.). *Paroxysmal* tachycardias, which start and stop abruptly, are caused by either a sudden burst of automaticity or the establishment of a reentry loop

---

*They are not uniformly retrograde, however.

TABLE I–2. Supraventricular Tachyarrhythmias (Classification).

  I. Sinus tachycardia
 II. Paroxysmal tachycardias
   A. Paroxysmal burst of automaticity
     Paroxysmal ectopic atrial tachycardia (PAT)
   B. Interatrial reentry loop
     1. "Benign slow PAT"
     2. Atrial flutter
   C. Large reentry loop involving the A–V node (and occasionally a bundle of Kent)
     Reentrant supraventricular tachycardia (RSVT)
III. Nonparoxysmal tachycardias
   A. Nonparoxysmal ectopic atrial tachycardia (NPAT, "PAT with block")
   B. Nonparoxysmal junctional tachycardia (Accelerated junctional rhythm [AJR])
IV. Chaotic atrial mechanism
   A. Chaotic (multifocal) atrial tachycardia (CAT)
   B. Atrial fibrillation (AF)

("circus"). When *sustained,* they often respond to vagal maneuvers or DC cardioversion.* *Nonparoxysmal* tachycardias result from the gradual but progressive increase in the rate of discharge of an atrial or junctional pacemaker until it becomes the dominant rhythm. Vagal maneuvers and DC shock are ineffective in breaking the rhythm.** In addition, since most of these nonparoxysmal accelerations are caused by digitalis toxicity, DC shock may be quite dangerous.*** Finally, *chaotic atrial mechanisms* include multifocal atrial discharges and outright atrial fibrillation. The electrocardiographic and clinical features of all these rhythms are summarized in Table I–3.

During any rapid supraventricular arrhythmia, some or all of the QRS-complexes may develop a BBB pattern because of (1) functional aberration or (2) rate-related ("tachycardia-dependent") BBB. The diagnostic problem of tachyarrhythmias with widened QRS-complexes will be discussed in Section III. All supraventricular tachyarrhythmias may occur in both health and disease; none is specific for any form of heart disease. Hyperthyroidism must always be excluded in all cases, including, of course, unexplained sustained sinus tachycardia.

"Benign Slow Atrial Tachycardia"

This is an ectopic atrial rhythm, usually beginning as a PAC and occurring at rates between 90 and 140 bpm. The rate tends to be somewhat irregular, and the rhythm tends to spontaneously break after short periods of time. This rhythm, which starts and stops abruptly, also may be abolished by digitalis, propranolol, vagal maneuvers, and Type I antiarrhythmic drugs (quinidine, procainamide, disopyramide). The electrophysiologic mechanism is felt to be a reentry circuit within the atrium. In rare cases, the P-waves exactly resemble the sinus-P-waves in every lead; S–A nodal reentry is the postulated mechanism.

Paroxysmal Ectopic Atrial Tachycardia (PAT)

This rhythm probably represents the rapid firing of an ectopic atrial focus (although a mini-reentry circuit within the atrium cannot be excluded). It begins with a PAC and terminates abruptly. The P-waves have a constant, ectopic, non-retrograde morphology, and occur at a rate of 150 to 250 bpm (most are between 180 and

---

*If occurring in nonsustained, intermittent bursts, DC shock or vagal maneuvers are of no use.
**Vagal maneuvers will further increase the A–V block, however.
***Intractable ventricular fibrillation or flat line may result.

TABLE I-3. Supraventricular Tachyarrhythmias (Characteristics).

Rhythm	Sinus Tachy	PAT	"Benign Slow PAT"	Atrial Flutter	RSVT	NPAT	AJR	CAT	AF
Clinical Occurrence	Health/Disease	Health/Disease	Health/Disease	Usually Disease	Often Health	Usually Digtoxicity	Digtoxicity, Acute MI	COPD	Usually Disease
Heart Rate	100–200 (160 upper limit beyond age 50)	A 150–250 (most 180–220) V 80–250 (most 1:1)	90–140	A 250–350 (most 300) V 75–300* (most 150)	120–250 (most 150–220)	A 100–250 V 75–100 (2:1–4:1 common)	60–160 (rarely above)	A 120–250 V 100–250	A 300–600 V 30–300* (most 70–150)
Initiation	Gradual acceleration	PAC	PAC	PAC, AF	Prolonged A–V or V–A conduction	Gradual acceleration	Gradual acceleration	PAC	PAC, atrial flutter
Response to Vagal Maneuvers	May *slightly* slow	None, stop, ↓ vent. response	Usually stop	↓ vent. response	None, stop	↓ vent. response	None	Usually none	↓ vent. response
Response to Digitalis	Will slow *if due to heart failure*	Usually stop; ↓ vent. response	Usually stop	↓ vent. response**	Usually stop	(Contraindicated)	(Contraindicated if due to digitalis toxicity)	None, conversion to AF	↓ vent. response#
Therapy	*Treat underlying cause*	Vagal° digitalis propranolol Type I## verapamil	Vagal° digitalis propranolol Type I##	DC shock† rapid pacing digitalis†† propranolol verapamil Type I## [1,2]	Vagal° verapamil digitalis propranolol induced PAC or PVC DC shock† Lidocaine and/or Type I## (response to Lidocaine indicates presence of Kent bundle in reentry circuit)	Stop digitalis; replenish potassium (DC shock contraindicated)	Stop digitalis (if digtoxic) (No therapy if due to acute MI) (DC shock contraindicated if due to digtoxicity)	*Improve respiratory status;* digitalis	Digitalis†† DC shock† verapamil propranolol Type I## [1,2]

[1] W-P-W with heart rate 300 bpm: Immediate DC shock or lidocaine (if efficacious).

[2] *Never* use Type I agent alone (without digitalis) for conversion or chronic prophylaxis.

*Heart rate 250–300: Antegrade Kent bundle conduction present, or, in the case of atrial flutter with HR 220–250, presence of quinidine without digitalis.

**The ventricular response is often more difficult to slow than in AF.

#One does not expect the ventricular response to decrease below comparable sinus rate if sinus tachycardia were present (i.e., because of fever, hyperthyroidism, pulmonary embolism, etc.).

°Carotid massage, Tensilon, Valsalva, methoxamine (RSVT with low normal or low BP).

##Quinidine, procainamide, disopyramide.

†To be used only if rhythm is sustained.

††Tensilon may be used to acutely slow the ventricular response.

220 bpm). The atrial rate during PAT is usually *perfectly regular*. There is usually 1:1 conduction to the ventricles (atrial and ventricular rates equal with constant P–R interval), but the presence of heightened vagal tone or drugs (digitalis, propranolol) may decrease A–V conduction (various A–V Wenckebach ratios,* such as 8:7, 5:4, 4:3, etc.; 2:1, 3:1 or, rarely 4:1 block). PAT may be present in long runs which start and stop spontaneously. If sustained, however, when vagal maneuvers are applied (carotid massage, Tensilon, Valsalva, or raising of the blood pressure with pressors), any of the following responses may occur: (1) no response, (2) rhythm may break abruptly (the atrial rate may sometimes slow slightly before terminating), (3) atrial tachycardia persists, but there is a decrease in A–V conduction (3:2, 2:1, 3:1, etc.). Digitalis usually terminates the rhythm, but, occasionally is either completely unsuccessful or merely decreases A–V conduction. The same can be said for propranolol, but, in addition, the atrial rate may decrease. Type I antiarrhythmic agents may also decrease the atrial rate and/or terminate the arrhythmia. Verapamil decreases A–V conduction and occasionally terminates the arrhythmia.

Unlike sinus tachycardia, PAT is rarely interrupted by a PAC from another focus; in addition, as previously mentioned, the atrial rate is almost always *perfectly regular*. When the atrial rate is 150 to 180 bpm, and the P-wave morphology is such that they *could be* of sinus origin, the presence of PACs or a slightly phasically irregular atrial rate points to *marked sinus tachycardia* rather than PAT. In rare instances there is a "long-short" cycle-to-cycle variation in the atrial rate; the mechanism for such variation has been a subject for speculation, but remains unknown. Even more rarely, there may be a Wenckebach exit block between the ectopic focus and the atrium; in such cases, a regularly irregular ectopic P to P cycle length variation ("group beating") occurs.

Since PAT begins as a premature beat, the first and any number of subsequent QRSs may show BBB due to functional aberration. Before the onset, and following the termination of PAT, ectopic atrial beats from the same focus, occurring as either early beats (single PACs and salvoes) or late beats, are often present.

PAT is not indicative of digitalis toxicity.

---

*In an A–V Wenckebach period, there is progressive increase in the P–R interval, culminating in a single nonconducted P-wave. The ratio of Ps to QRSs is therefore 5:4, 4:3, etc. Wenckebach periods will be further discussed later in this Section, and at length in Section II.

Nonparoxysmal Ectopic Atrial Tachycardia (NPAT)

In contradistinction to true PAT, in which an ectopic atrial pacemaker has a sudden burst of rapid firing, in nonparoxysmal atrial tachycardia (NPAT), an ectopic atrial focus becomes progressively accelerated until it becomes the dominant pacemaker of the heart. The cause is almost always digitalis toxicity. Because the digitalis decreases A–V nodal conduction, significant A–V block (2:1, 3:1, or worse) always accompanies the accelerated atrial rhythm; hence, the popular misnomer, "PAT with block." The A–V conduction ratio may be constant or variable. The atrial rate is 100 to 250 bpm (most are between 150 and 200 bpm). The P-wave morphology is ectopic and nonretrograde; in a number of cases, the ectopic P-wave resembles the sinus-P except for relatively subtle differences, or differences noted in only some of the leads. The atrial rate is perfectly regular, although in rare instances "long-short" cycle variation of the P–P interval occurs.

The diagnosis of this rhythm may at times be easily missed. Occasionally, the P-waves are of extremely small amplitude, apparent in only one or two of the 12 ECG leads. The P-waves may be of reasonable size, but the second, nonconducted P-wave in 2:1 block may be buried in the preceding ST-segment or T-wave; if BBB is present, it may even be completely masked by the widened QRS. It is, therefore, always good practice, whenever dealing with apparent sinus or ectopic atrial rhythm of 150 bpm or less, to take half the obvious P–P interval and in every lead see where the *second* P-wave would occur if the true atrial rate were *double* the apparent rate. If there is deformity of the QRS-T at that site, one may indeed be dealing with NPAT with 2:1 block (or, possibly atrial flutter if the atrial rate is 260 or more bpm). In addition, vagal maneuvers, such as carotid massage, greatly increase the A–V block, permitting the underlying atrial activity to be seen. In cases of apparent "ectopic atrial rhythm," if the second P-wave would fall completely within a QRS widened by BBB, one should definitely obtain a long rhythm strip and do vagal maneuvers in an attempt to unmask extra P-waves.

When the correct diagnosis has been made, the withholding of digitalis and administration of potassium cause the firing of the ectopic atrial focus to gradually decelerate and finally disappear. During the tenure of this rhythm, vagal maneuvers merely cause an increase in the A–V block. Since the rhythm represents a *gradual* acceleration of an ectopic focus of automaticity, these maneuvers are ineffective in abolishing it. This rhythm is non-paroxysmal and it is never seen on a rhythm strip to start or stop. DC shock and, of course, digitalis are contraindicated in digitalis toxicity.* In addition, those rare cases of chronic non-digitalis-toxic NPAT tend to be refractory to cardioversion. In NPAT with advanced or complete heart block, and a slow heart rate and/or unresponsiveness to atropine, a temporary transvenous pacemaker must be inserted. If antiarrhythmic drugs or DC shock are required for ventricular arrhythmias, a flat line may result if a pacemaker is not employed.

When Is an Ectopic Atrial Tachycardia a Digitalis-Toxic Rhythm?

Atrial tachycardia with 1:1 or close to 1:1 conduction (i.e., Wenckebach 3:2, 4:3 or better) is PAT, and is not digitalis-toxic. Atrial tachycardia with 2:1, 3:1 or worse conduction may be:

1. Digitalis-toxic NPAT
2. Non-digitalis-toxic chronic NPAT (these rare cases are seen in patients with chronic heart failure with marked enlargement of both the left atrium and ventricle)
3. Recurrent true PAT, with block caused by *therapeutic doses* of digitalis and/or propranolol—these are not digitalis-toxic.

Since digitalis-toxic NPAT with block is by far most likely, *atrial tachycardia with 2:1 or worse block should be considered digitalis-toxic until proven otherwise.* Low or absent serum digitalis level with normal serum potassium level, or a history of recurrent PAT, with previous ECGs to document the similar P-wave morphology and/or previously obtained therapeutic A–V block in the case of (3), are needed to rule out digitalis-toxic NPAT. Chronic non-digitalis-toxic NPAT is diagnosed by exclusion. Finally, NPAT is a *nonparoxysmal* arrhythmia; if the atrial tachycardia is observed on the rhythm strip to start and stop, it is clearly a *paroxysmal* arrhythmia (i.e., PAT).

Atrial Flutter

Atrial flutter is characterized by an atrial rate of 250 to 350 bpm (most are exactly 300 bpm). The ventricular response is frequently 2:1 (i.e., heart rate 150 bpm), but other conducting ratios (4:1, variable) commonly occur. For some reason, odd-number conducting ratios (3:1, 5:1, etc.) are rare.* The flutter waves may resemble small, discrete P-waves, or may appear, particularly in Leads II, III and aVF, as a regular "sawtooth" baseline. Occasionally, the flutter waves are low amplitude, and are visible in only one or two leads. *Coarse atrial fibrillation* (to be discussed later) may resemble atrial flutter, but, in the latter, the flutter wave rate and morphology are *perfectly uniform,* while, in atrial fibrillation, some variation is always found. Since the flutter waves may appear as discrete, small P-waves, it is possible to misdiagnose atrial flutter as sinus tachycardia if the second flutter wave is overlooked. Atrial flutter must always be considered when faced with a supraventricular rhythm at a heart rate of 150 bpm, since 300 bpm is the most frequent flutter rate, and 2:1 the most common conducting ratio. As always, one divides the obvious P–P interval in half to see where a second P-wave (or flutter wave) would occur, and whether the QRS-T is indeed deformed at that site. Whenever there is a change in P-wave morphology (especially to narrower, smaller-amplitude P-waves), accompanied by a decrease in P–R interval and an increase in the heart rate to 130 to 160 bpm, atrial flutter must be considered. In addition to looking for a second P-wave in a given lead, one should carefully search all 12 leads for flutter activity. Whenever one is faced with a tachycardia (with narrow or wide QRS-complexes) in which, although no discrete P-waves are seen, there is a sharp angularity to the QRS-T complexes, atrial flutter must be considered (see ECG III–66).

As previously mentioned, the heart rate during atrial flutter may be regular (e.g., 2:1, 4:1 response) or irregular (variable conduction). If the average heart rate is above 100 bpm, the ventricular response is said to be *rapid, moderate* between 60 and 100 bpm, and *slow* under 60 bpm. Most undigitalized patients have a rapid response. If atrial flutter is suspected, a long rhythm strip should be obtained and vagal maneuvers, which usually slow the ventricular response, should be employed to unmask the underlying flutter activity.

Flutter waves may deform the initial and terminal portions of the QRS-complex to produce the illusion of pathologic Q-waves or deep, terminal S-waves, respectively. Occasionally, the angular sawtooth flutter waves may deform both the QRS-complex and ST-segment to produce the illusion of an acute myocardial infarction; this is particu-

---

*DC shock must, of course, be used to treat sustained ventricular tachycardia, unresponsive to drugs, or ventricular fibrillation.

---

*Atrial flutter with an odd-number conducting ratio probably represents bilevel block within the A–V node. See Section II.

larly true in the inferior leads, where the QRS-complexes may be small and the flutter waves particularly prominent.

Type I antiarrhythmic drugs and propranolol tend to slow the rate of the flutter waves; digitalis may slightly increase it. Unlike digitalis and propranolol, the Type I drugs do not slow A–V nodal conduction; in fact, they may slightly enhance it by their vagolytic effect. Patients taking Type I agents alone, without benefit of digitalis or propranolol, may, if they go into atrial flutter, have a decreased flutter rate of 220 to 250 bpm *with 1:1 A–V conduction.* This rapid heart rate is, of course, extremely dangerous, and may precipitate hypotension, heart failure, or ischemia.

Atrial flutter may occur in paroxysms initiated by one or more PACs. *Atrial fibrillation,* to be discussed next, may spontaneously change to atrial flutter and *vice versa.* The first one or more QRSs of a paroxysm, or, one or more rapidly occurring beats during sustained atrial flutter with a variable response, may show functional aberration.

A ventricular response of 300 or more bpm implies that A–V conduction is bypassing the delay of the A–V node (and is, in fact, *via* a bundle of Kent).* In this case the QRS morphology is bizarre, since the ventricles are activated in an abnormal sequence originating from the site of exit of the Kent bundle in the myocardium. The Wolff-Parkinson-White (W-P-W) syndrome, in which antegrade (atrium to ventricle) Kent bundle conduction occurs, will be discussed in Sections III and IV.

Digitalis, propranolol, and Type I antiarrhythmic agents occasionally abolish atrial flutter, but in most cases, the flutter remains or is converted to atrial fibrillation. In many cases rapid atrial pacing may capture and break the flutter ("entrainment"). Digitalis frequently does not slow the ventricular response in atrial flutter as easily or as well as in atrial fibrillation, probably because there are fewer impulses decrementally conducting and colliding in the A–V node. For this reason, many cardiologists prefer to initially convert sustained atrial flutter with DC shock or rapid pacing entrainment, rather than attempting slowing or conversion with digitalis. When digitalis is contemplated, good slowing of the heart rate with vagal maneuvers usually predicts good slowing with digitalis. Rapid slowing of the heart rate may be achieved with verapamil, propranolol, or Tensilon.

---

*Under these circumstances, emergency DC shock is required if lidocaine fails to slow the rate. Digitalis may *increase* Kent bundle conduction in some patients.

Is a Supraventricular Tachycardia with an Atrial Rate of 250 bpm PAT or Atrial Flutter?

With an atrial rate of 250 bpm, the rhythm could represent either PAT or atrial flutter. If the classic "sawtooth" activity is seen, the rhythm is, of course, atrial flutter. Most flutter rates are 300 bpm; if Type I antiarrhythmics or propranolol are being taken, a rate of 250 bpm may result. On the other hand, 250 bpm tends to be the *fastest* possible rate for PAT; the above medications also often *slow* the atrial rate. Therefore, *if these drugs are being taken,* a rate of 250 bpm most likely represents atrial flutter; a widened QRS or Q–T interval helps to confirm the drug effect. If no such drugs are being taken, or if the medications are unknown but no QRS-T effect is seen, the rhythm is more likely to be PAT. Finally, if the P-wave morphology is identical to that of isolated PACs previously present, the diagnosis is PAT.

Atrial Fibrillation (AF)

Atrial fibrillation (AF) results from complete disorganization of atrial activity. The ECG shows no discrete atrial activity; rather, the baseline shows irregular, nonuniform undulations. At times these undulations may be quite coarse, and may mimic discrete P-waves (atrial flutter or PAT). However, careful examination of the rhythm strip reveals nonuniformity of the atrial rate and contour, indicative of AF. In well-digitalized and frankly digitalis-toxic patients, the AF baseline undulations often become less coarse, and may finally disappear altogether, leaving a completely smooth baseline.

Since, during AF, the A–V node is bombarded with 300 to 600 impulses per minute, with both irregular bombardment and unpredictable fade-out and collisions within the A–V node, the ventricular response is *irregularly irregular.* However, during both rapid and slow ventricular responses, and, occasionally, even during a moderate response (as with atrial flutter, 60 to 100 bpm is considered a moderate response), the QRS cycle-to-cycle variation may be minimal. If many cycles are carefully measured, a small degree of variation becomes apparent.

AF, like PAT and flutter, may be paroxysmal or sustained. It is usually initiated by one or more PACs, although it may result from conversion of atrial flutter or chaotic atrial tachycardia (to be shortly discussed). The first one or more beats of a short paroxysm of AF, or, if sustained, one or more rapidly occurring beats during the course of

AF may show functional aberration; in the latter case, the differentiation from a run of ventricular tachycardia must be made (this will be thoroughly discussed in Section III).

Regularization of the heart rate in the presence of AF means that complete block of conduction through the A–V node has occurred, with the resulting rhythm coming from a regularly discharging infranodal pacemaker (in the junction, or, occasionally, in the bundle branches). A *regularly irregular* rhythm similarly implies complete A–V nodal block; in this case, however, there is additional block of Wenckebach type between the junction and the ventricle. The cause of both the above situations is almost always digitalis toxicity (and, *very rarely*, acute inferior wall myocardial infarction). Junctional rhythm will be further discussed later.

As with atrial flutter, digitalis, propranolol, and vagal maneuvers slow the ventricular response, sometimes markedly. Digitalis, propranolol, and Type I antiarrhythmic drugs may also completely abolish AF, resulting in restoration of sinus rhythm.

When digitalis is employed to slow the ventricular response, one titrates the drug with the heart rate, usually aiming for 70 to 90 bpm. It is important to remember that digitalis *therapeutically* never slows the heart rate below the comparable sinus rate, if the patient were in sinus rhythm. If the patient would have had a sinus tachycardia of 110 to 120 bpm because of fever, thyrotoxicosis, pulmonary embolism, etc., digitalis cannot be expected to slow the ventricular response to AF below that range. Conversely, if the ventricular response increases in a previously well-digitalized patient, a search must be made for an underlying cause. In an acute situation in which a patient presents with atrial fibrillation or flutter with a rapid response, and immediate cardioversion is not desired, the rate may be rapidly slowed with Tensilon (intravenous bolus followed by constant infusion), or, if there is no heart failure or hypotension, with intravenous propranolol. In the absence of non-arrhythmia related hypotension or severe heart failure, intravenous verapamil may prove to be the drug of choice.

In those patients with W-P-W who have Kent bundles capable of repetitive rapid antegrade conduction, the ventricular response to AF may reach or exceed 300 bpm, as with atrial flutter. Again, the QRS-complexes are bizarre, since antegrade A–V conduction is *via* the Kent bundle. DC shock is required for emergency cardioversion if lidocaine fails to slow Kent bundle conduction. Digi-talis may *increase* Kent bundle conduction in some patients.

Although well-digitalized, with a moderate ventricular response, most patients in atrial fibrillation demonstrate a wide range of heart rates on 24-hour Holter monitoring (tending to be slow during sleep, faster during daytime activities). Most un-digitalized patients have an average ventricular response of 120 to 160 bpm, although, as with atrial flutter, younger patients with heightened vagal tone, and older patients with A–V nodal disease, may have moderate, even slow ventricular responses. *The initial ventricular response (even if slow) does not predict the degree of subsequent slowing by digitalis.** However, as with atrial flutter, atrial fibrillation with a slow response in an elderly patient not taking digitalis may require a pacemaker if spontaneous or digitalis-induced, lengthy, symptomatic pauses occur, or if heart failure is present.

Chaotic Atrial Tachycardia (Multifocal Atrial Tachycardia)

This rhythm, usually seen in patients with pulmonary disease, most often while in respiratory distress, is characterized by an irregular atrial rate of 120 to 250 bpm. Each of the P-waves has a different morphology; the P–R intervals also show variation. A–V conduction is frequently 1:1, but 2:1 and variable conduction also occur. Chaotic atrial tachycardia (CAT) is usually sustained, but long runs of CAT separated by a few sinus beats (generally sinus tachycardia) may be seen. CAT is often mistaken for AF, since the ever-changing P-waves may be mistaken for undulations in the baseline. Careful examination of the ECG reveals discrete P-waves. As with AF, some of the more rapidly occurring beats may show functional aberration. Digitalis may convert the rhythm to either sinus (tachycardia with frequent PACs) or AF; however, amelioration of the patient's respiratory status is the definitive therapy.

Reentrant Supraventricular Tachycardia (RSVT) ("Reciprocating Tachycardia," "A–V Nodal Tachycardia")

In this rhythm, a reentry loop becomes established, usually within the A–V node.** In most individuals, the A–V node has multiple physiologic, though anatomically indistinct, pathways. These are usually conceptualized as dual, "alpha"

---

*As with atrial flutter, good slowing with carotid massage or Tensilon predicts good slowing with digitalis; conversely, the presence of digitalis potentiates the response to vagal maneuvers.

**Occasionally, reentry within the atria may occur.

and "beta," or "fast" and "slow," pathways. The slow pathway has slow antegrade conduction, but a relatively short antegrade refractory period. The fast pathway has more rapid antegrade conduction and a relatively short retrograde refractory period. Under certain conditions, an antegrade impulse may be blocked in the fast pathway while conducting slowly down the slow pathway. Given a critical degree of slowing, an impulse may arrive at the lower reaches of the A–V node* *via* the slow pathway and find the fast pathway already recovered and able to conduct in the retrograde direction. The impulse then travels up the fast pathway to the upper reaches of the A–V node, from where it may (1) stimulate the atrium in retrograde fashion, producing an *atrial echo* (retrograde-P-wave derived from original antegrade conduction), and/or (2) find the slow pathway able to conduct in the antegrade direction, thus beginning another reentry loop. If conditions permit, the loop tachycardia continues, each loop giving off an atrial echo from the upper portion and a *ventricular echo* (antegrade stimulation of the ventricle derived from previous retrograde conduction) from the lower portion; a ventricular echo is a supraventricular QRS-complex, similar in morphology to the previous sinus beats, unless widened by functional aberration. The tachyarrhythmia thus formed abruptly terminates when (1) critical A–V nodal slowing occurs, causing the impulse to "peter out" in the loop, and/or (2) part of the loop circuit is rendered refractory by another critically timed impulse (spontaneously occurring or pacing-induced premature atrial or ventricular beat) which enters the circuit, preempting and, thus, blocking the loop impulse. In the dog, the atrium is believed to be an integral part of the reentrant loop; in humans, sufficient clinical examples of the atrium's not being part of the circuit exist (see ECGs I–55 and I–59), so that the scheme presented in Figure I–2 is probably a more appropriate model. In about 20% of patients having clinically typical RSVT, the retrograde portion of the loop is not in the A–V node, but, rather *via retrograde conduction through a bundle of Kent*. In many of these cases, the Kent bundle is incapable of antegrade conduction, so the W-P-W syndrome is absent during sinus rhythm. That an accessory A–V connection (Kent bundle) is utilized for the return pathway may be proved by intracardiac electrophysiologic studies. In reentrant arrhythmias utilizing a Kent bundle, the atrium must of necessity be part of the reentrant loop (see Figure

I–3). In a small minority of patients with W-P-W, the reentrant loop involves *antegrade* Kent bundle conduction (with retrograde return *via* the A–V node); in these cases, the QRS-complexes are bizarre (see ECG III–73); such RSVTs may mimic ventricular tachycardia. Fortunately, most Kent bundles are incapable of conducting rapidly repetitive impulses in the antegrade direction, so this type of RSVT, as well as AF and atrial flutter with heart rates of 300 bpm, are all rare.

The usual type of RSVT (reentry within the A–V node or utilizing retrograde Kent bundle conduction) is characterized by a regular narrow-QRS tachycardia at a rate of 120 to 250 bpm (most are 180 to 220 bpm). Retrograde-P-waves may be present; if so, they tend to occur during the first half of electrical diastole, that is, from the end of the QRS to a point approximately midway between QRSs. Frequently the retrograde-Ps are absent, presumably buried within the QRS-complexes. When present, there is one retrograde-P for every QRS, except in those rare, interesting cases where retrograde activation of the atrium by the loop transiently fails; the retrograde-P-wave is intermittently absent.* In yet rarer cases, there may be transient complete block in the upper portion of the A–V node, above the site of the reentry loop. Sinus-P-waves, dissociated from the RSVT, may occur (see ECG II–44).

As previously discussed, the prerequisite for A–V nodal reentry (that is, the bouncing back of an impulse) is critical slowing of A–V conduction. This may occur in cases of original antegrade conduction delay, as previously discussed; it may also occur in cases of original *retrograde* conduction delay. The antecedent causes of both antegrade and retrograde A–V conduction delay which may initiate reentry are summarized in Table I–4. Since the beat initiating an RSVT is an early beat, and the RSVT itself is rapid and regular, anywhere from one to all of the QRSs may have functional aberration.

Vagal maneuvers have two possible responses: (1) immediate and sudden breaking of the rhythm, or, (2) no response. Since the arrhythmia is caused by a constantly active reentry loop, A–V conduction cannot significantly slow without cessation of the arrhythmia. When the rhythm does break, either spontaneously or following vagal maneuvers, a slight degree of slowing of the last two to three

---

*The so-called "final common pathway," where slow and fast pathways are joined.

*If no retrograde-P-waves are present, A–V nodal reentry is most likely; if they are visible beyond the QRS, the reentry circuit may or may not involve a concealed Kent bundle for the retrograde pathway; if they are intermittently absent the reentry loop is located exclusively in the A–V node.

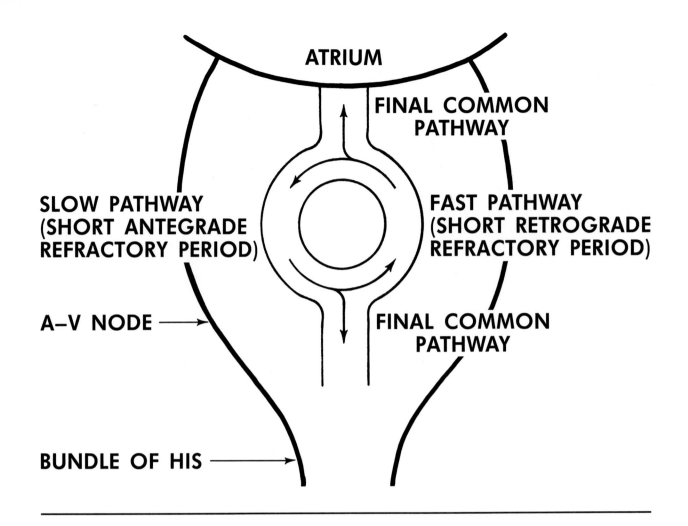

ATRIUM

FINAL COMMON PATHWAY

SLOW PATHWAY
(SHORT ANTEGRADE
REFRACTORY PERIOD)

FAST PATHWAY
(SHORT RETROGRADE
REFRACTORY PERIOD)

A–V NODE

FINAL COMMON
PATHWAY

BUNDLE OF HIS

SEQUENCE OF EVENTS

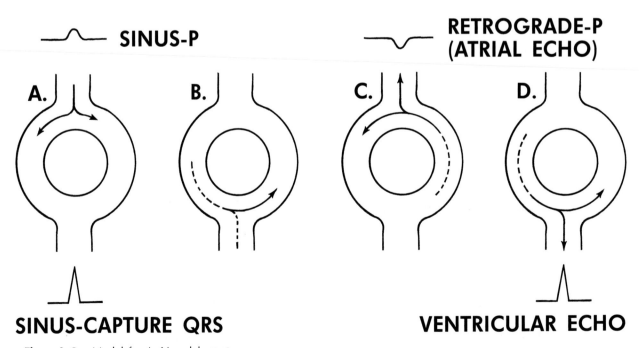

SINUS-P

RETROGRADE-P
(ATRIAL ECHO)

A.   B.   C.   D.

SINUS-CAPTURE QRS

VENTRICULAR ECHO

Figure I–2. Model for A–V nodal reentry.

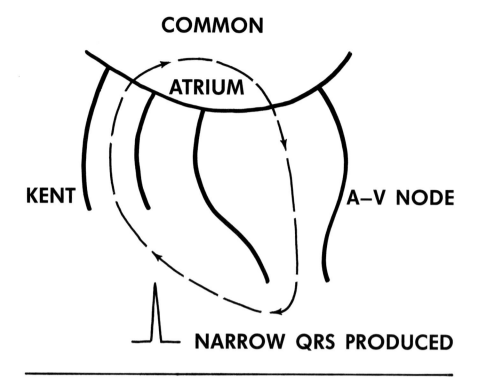

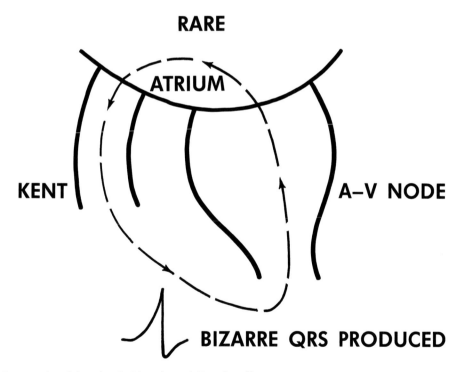

Figure I–3. Reentry involving the A–V node and Kent bundle.

beats is often noted. Digitalis is often effective in terminating the arrhythmia. Verapamil is also frequently effective, and may prove to be the drug of choice, should vagal maneuvers fail to terminate the tachycardia. In addition, intravenous lidocaine or procainamide may be useful in breaking an RSVT involving a Kent bundle in the reentry circuit; the latter may also be effective in some A–V nodal reentrant tachycardias. Finally, an RSVT may be broken by interrupting the reentry circuit using critically timed paced beats, singly or in salvoes.

TABLE I–4.   Initiation of A–V Nodal Reentry.

I. Antegrade A–V nodal delay
  A. PAC with 1° A–V block
  B. A–V Wenckebach period (SR or PAT)
  C. 1° A–V block in a sinus beat closely following a PJC, PVC,* junctional escape beat, or ventricular-paced beat
II. Retrograde A–V nodal delay
  A. V–A Wenckebach period (junctional or ventricular rhythms, including ventricular tachycardia)
  B. Prolonged V–A conduction from a PJC, PVC, or ventricular-paced beat

*Premature ventricular beat

It is important to remember that in RSVT a retrograde-P-wave does not "make" the subsequent QRS, or *vice versa;* both are "spin-offs" from the reentry loop.

What Happens to the Sinus Upon Termination of PAT, RSVT, or Paroxysms of AF or Flutter?

There may be a pause of 1 to 3 sec. until sinus rhythm resumes, especially if vagal maneuvers were employed to break PAT or RSVT. Following the first sinus escape beat, a normal sinus promptly warms up, so that normal sinus rhythm is quickly resumed. (Again, lingering vagal effect from digitalis and/or maneuvers may produce transient S–A or A–V Wenckebach periods.) In cases of a sick sinus mechanism, following cessation of the tachyarrhythmia, prolonged periods of asystole, both before and after the first escape beat, may ensue.

A–V Dissociation

During embryonic life, as each region of the heart is formed, the heart beat is controlled by pacemaker cells within that region. Beginning with the ventricles, then the atria, and finally the sinus area, as each new region is successively added, its pacemaker cells, having a faster rate of discharge than those in the lower region, control the heart beat. The final region, high in the right atrium, establishes the S–A node as the dominant pacemaker of the heart. The centers of automaticity of the lower regions remain as a hierarchy of subsidiary latent pacemakers, whose discharges are usually continuously suppressed by the faster sinus.* These subsidiary pacemakers and their usual escape rates are given in Table I–5. A latent focus may become the dominant pacemaker under three conditions: (1) if the sinus rate falls below that of the subsidiary pacemaker, permitting the latter to escape; (2) if the subsidiary pacemaker accelerates to a rate faster than the sinus; (3) if heart block develops, so that the sinus impulse cannot reach the subsidiary pacemaker (in such cases, the *highest* (fastest) pacemaker located *below* the level of block takes over). During periods of *A–V dissociation* the atria and ventricles are under control of separate pacemakers; that is, the atria by the sinus or an

*Occasionally, the sinus fails to enter a subsidiary pacemaker ("entrance block"), permitting it to reach threshold and discharge (i.e., escape); a *parasystole* is said to result.

TABLE I–5.   Hierarchy of Cardiac Pacemakers.

	Pacemaker	Location	Name of Escape Rhythm	Usual Escape Rate	Name of Accelerated Rhythm	Rate of Accelerated Rhythm
Primary (Dominant) Pacemakers	Sinus	S–A node	SR	60–100	Sinus tachycardia	> 100
	Ectopic atrial	Atria	Ectopic atrial rhythm	50–80	NPAT	A 100–250 V 75–100
Subsidiary (Latent) Pacemakers	Junctional	N–H region of A–V node, His bundle	Junctional rhythm	35–60	AJR	> 60
	Subjunctional	Proximal bundle branch fascicles	Subjunctional rhythm	30–50	ASJR	> 60
	Ventricular	Ventricular Purkinje network	Idioventricular rhythm	0–35	Accelerated idioventricular rhythm	35–100
					Ventricular tachycardia	100–250

TABLE I−6. Causes of A−V Dissociation.

1. Slowing of the primary (sinus or atrial) pacemaker
2. Acceleration of a subsidiary (junctional, subjunctional, or ventricular) pacemaker
3. Advanced or complete A−V block
4. Any combination of the above

ectopic atrial pacemaker, and the ventricles by a junctional or ventricular pacemaker. If occasional capture of the ventricles by the atria (i.e., antegrade capture), or capture of the atria by the junction or ventricles (i.e., retrograde capture) occurs, *incomplete* A−V dissociation is said to be present; when no such captures occur, the dissociation is said to be *complete*. The causes of A−V dissociation are identical to those which cause a subsidiary pacemaker to become dominant, and are summarized in Table I−6. As can be seen, *A−V block is but one of the causes of A−V dissociation; the two are not synonymous.*

On first glance of a rhythm strip in which A−V dissociation is present, one sees P-waves with an inconstant relationship to the QRSs; the former may "march through" the latter. If the QRS-complexes are regular, the ventricles are being driven by junctional rhythm if they are supraventricular, or by ventricular rhythm (idioventricular or ventricular tachycardia) if wide and bizarre.

If junctional rhythm is present and there are occasional *early supraventricular* QRSs, the differential diagnosis of the latter includes: (1) antegrade captures by the sinus or atrium; (2) ventricular echoes; or, (3) PJCs. Each *sinus capture* is preceded by a *sinus-P-wave* having a physiologically feasible P−R interval (0.12 to 0.60 sec.); the closer the P-wave to the preceding junctional QRS, the longer the P−R interval, since the conducting system is more refractory.* Each *ventricular echo* is preceded by a *retrograde-P-wave;* as with antegrade captures, the length of the P−R interval is inversely proportional to the preceding R−P interval. Examination of the preceding two or more junctional beats reveals a *V−A Wenckebach period* (i.e., progressive delay of retrograde conduction through the A−V node), characterized by increasing R to retrograde-P intervals. In this situation, that is, junctional rhythm with V−A Wenckebach periods and ventricular echoes, *no* A−V dissociation is present if there are no sinus or ectopic atrial P-waves, since *all* the retrograde-P-waves and QRSs are related to each other in an organized, regularly repetitive,

though inconstant fashion.* If, following a dropped retrograde-P-wave, the sinus escapes for one or more beats which are unrelated to the subsequent junctional QRSs, incomplete A−V dissociation (or, put another way, periods of A−V dissociation at the time of the sinus-P-waves) is said to be present. If no sinus-P-waves are present, the sinus rate can be inferred to be slower than the longest retrograde-P to retrograde-P interval.

Early supraventricular beats interrupting junctional rhythm may also rarely be PJCs. The diagnosis is made by exclusion, that is, by the absence of P-waves preceding the early QRSs. However, one must be quite careful that a preceding P-wave is not buried in the previous QRS-T. In addition, the early QRS may be a ventricular echo despite the absence of a preceding retrograde-P-wave (i.e., the retrogradely conducted junctional impulse reached the upper region of the A−V node, and, despite being unable to reach the atrium, was conducted back down the other of the dual pathways to make the ventricular echo).** This and other examples of *concealed conduction* will be discussed in Section IV.

Suppose there is an atrial rhythm (including SR) with at least some P-waves unrelated to the QRS-complexes and, therefore, an *irregular* heart rate (i.e., varying R−R intervals). The junctional escape beats (whether escaping at their normal rate or at an accelerated rate) are identified as follows: by definition, all junctional escape beats terminate the *longest* R−R intervals. Measure all the R−R intervals: (1) Suppose there are two or more that are equal in length, and are longer than the others. The beats terminating these equal and longest R−R intervals are junctional escape beats if they have an inconsistent relationship to their respective preceding P-waves (i.e., since each is related to the preceding QRS-complex and *not* to the preceding P-wave, A−V dissociation is present), or if the preceding P−R intervals are equal, but not feasible for capture. All of the QRSs terminating the shorter R−R intervals therefore represent sinus captures. (2) If the longest R−R interval occurs only *once*, the QRS terminating that interval may or may not represent a junctional escape beat. If the atrial rate is faster than the ventricular rate, the

---

*For P-waves well beyond the preceding T-wave, the conducting system is usually considered to have completely recovered, so that the P−R intervals for such beats are usually constant.

---

*If the retrograde-P-waves are *perfectly regular*, the rhythm is really A−V dissociation between an ectopic atrial rhythm and a junctional escape rhythm with occasional antegrade captures. In a V−A Wenckebach period, a *progressive decrease* of the retrograde P−P intervals precedes the ventricular echo or dropped retrograde-P-wave.
**Here again, preceding V−A Wenckebach conduction is evident.

QRS is a junctional escape beat if it is not preceded by a P-wave having a feasible (0.12 to 0.60 sec.) capture interval.* When the atrial rate exceeds the ventricular rate, there must be some degree of A–V block with variable A–V conduction, since the R–R intervals vary; in this case, when the QRS terminating a single longest R–R interval is preceded by a feasible P-wave, one cannot differentiate between a junctional escape beat and a sinus capture following higher-grade A–V block.** If the ventricular rate exceeds the atrial rate, the beat terminating a single longest R–R interval is a junctional escape if it is not preceded by a feasible P-wave.

When faced with a supraventricular rhythm with A–V dissociation, the key question is: What is the cause(s) of the A–V dissociation? Is the sinus simply slower than the junctional rate? (If the latter is adequate and unaccelerated, the rhythm is clinically benign.) Is the junction accelerated? (This is digitalis-toxic until proven otherwise.) Is A–V block present? (This may require a pacemaker, or other therapy.) Remember, there may be *more than one cause* for A–V dissociation.

To ascertain the cause(s), first identify the junctional escape beats, as outlined above. Measurement of the R–R interval terminating in a junctional escape beat provides the junctional rate. If 35 to 60 bpm, it is normal; if 60 or more bpm, it is accelerated. Next, compare the sinus rate to the junctional rate. Finally, ascertain whether A–V block is present. To do this, answer the following question: Are there any P-waves in a position to capture (i.e., produce QRS-complexes), which do not? Remember the following four "rules of thumb": (1) a P-wave must be beyond the T-wave of the preceding beat in order to be *expected* to capture (although earlier P-waves, within the ST-T complex *may be able* to do so); (2) the range of feasible P–R intervals for capture is about 0.12 to 0.60 sec. (i.e., if a P-wave beyond the T is followed after 0.60 sec. by a QRS, that QRS cannot be considered a capture; if a QRS occurs within 0.12 sec. following a sinus-P-wave, it should ordinarily not be considered a capture); (3) if several sinus captures whose P-waves occur *well beyond* the preceding T are identified, and are found to have a constant capture P–R interval of a certain amount, say, 0.18 sec., then, in a test situation, a QRS fol-

lowing a P-wave by less than 0.18 sec. should not be considered a capture; (4) if the atrial rate is rapid (greater than 100 bpm),* it may at times be impossible to determine *which* P-wave is capturing—a P-wave may be followed by a QRS after a P–R interval considered too short for capture, but the P–R interval may be feasible if measured back from the QRS to the *second* preceding P-wave. Occasionally, either of *two* P-waves could have produced the capture. Following the above rules, if P-waves which ought to capture are found not to do so, an element of A–V block (advanced or complete) is present. *If no captures are found, but no P-waves are in a position feasible for capture, the presence of A–V block cannot be ascertained.* In addition, if a P-wave beyond the preceding T is followed by a junctional escape beat after an interval of 0.12 to about 0.40 sec., it is possible that the P-wave could have captured with a slightly longer P–R interval, but was preempted by the junctional escape beat. The longer the P-to-junctional-QRS interval, the less likely is this possibility. Furthermore, if definite captures are present and have a P–R interval shorter than the P-to-junctional-QRS interval under consideration, this possibility is ruled out.

Occasionally, despite complete A–V dissociation, the sinus and junctional rates are nearly equal, with the QRS-complexes following the P-waves by an interval within the feasible capture range ("isorhythmic dissociation"); careful examination of a long rhythm strip is required to demonstrate an inconstant relationship between the two. If, under these circumstances, the interval between the P and QRS never exceeds 0.60 sec., the presence of A–V block cannot be ascertained, although the longer the P–R interval, the greater the probability of block.

In the absence of A–V block, a normal or accelerated junction ought never appear as long as the sinus rate exceeds the junctional rate. The exception to this rule occurs when a "full compensatory pause" occurs following a premature junctional or ventricular beat, or when the sinus is reset following a conducted or nonconducted PAC. Under such circumstances, an *accelerated junctional escape beat* (i.e., having an escape time of less than 1.0 sec., corresponding to a sustained escape rate of more than 60 bpm) may be unmasked, indicating digitalis toxicity long before A–V block and further junctional acceleration become manifest as *accelerated junctional rhythm* (AJR) and A–V dissociation.

---

*When the atrial rate is rapid, the *second* preceding P-wave may be feasible for capture, even if the *immediately* preceding P is not.

**If there is advanced A–V block with one or more fixed conducting ratios (e.g., 2:1), a beat terminating a single longest R–R interval is probably, though not definitely, a capture if the preceding P-wave has a P–R interval identical to that of the other captures.

---

*This holds true for sinus tachycardia, atrial tachycardia (PAT, NPAT), and atrial flutter.

Junctional Rhythm and Accelerated Junctional Rhythm; Subjunctional Rhythm and Accelerated Subjunctional Rhythm

Junctional rhythm originates in the pacemaker cells of the "N–H" region of the A–V node and in the bundle of His; the resulting QRS-complexes are supraventricular (narrow, unless altered by BBB, etc.). Subjunctional rhythm, though not, strictly speaking, supraventricular, is clinically and physiologically akin to junctional rhythm, and the subsequent discussion is equally applicable to both.*

The normal junctional escape rate is 35 to 60 bpm. In *accelerated junctional rhythm* (AJR) the rate exceeds 60 bpm (usual range: 60 to 120 bpm; rarely, as high as 160 bpm). The causes of junctional acceleration are listed in order of decreasing frequency in Table I–7; digitalis toxicity and acute myocardial infarction head the list. Unless another cause is obvious, junctional acceleration (manifested as either an accelerated junctional escape beat or AJR) *should be considered due to digitalis toxicity until proven otherwise.* Since AJR represents a gradual (nonparoxysmal) acceleration of a latent pacemaker, vagal maneuvers, drugs and DC shock are ineffective in terminating it. Digitalis and DC shock are, of course, contraindicated in the presence of digitalis toxicity.** If complete heart block (heart block with no capture) is present, and there is no improvement of conduction with atropine, a temporary transvenous pacemaker is required unless the junction is significantly accelerated (greater than 70 bpm). Should antiarrhythmic therapy be subsequently required, a slow, normal, or only mildly accelerated junction may become depressed; prolonged periods of asystole may re-

*Subjunctional rhythm arises in the proximal bundle branches; the resulting QRS-complexes have the appropriate BBB pattern. For example, if it arises in the posterior fascicle of the left bundle, the QRS has a RBBB + left anterior hemiblock pattern.
**DC shock may, of course, be required to convert sustained ventricular tachycardia unresponsive to drugs, or ventricular fibrillation.

TABLE I–7.   Causes of Junctional Acceleration.

1. Digitalis toxicity
2. Acute myocardial infarction
3. Catecholamine administration
4. Hypermetabolic state (hyperthyroidism, pheochromocytoma)
5. Open heart surgery (early post-op period)
6. Cardiac trauma
7. Atropine administration (transient rate increase)
8. Exercise (patients with congenital heart block with a high junctional pacemaker)

sult. Therapy consists of withholding digitalis and replenishing serum potassium if digitalis-toxic. Otherwise there is no specific therapy.

At any given time, the junctional escape rate is usually constant. Slight differences between escape rates of single beats, as well as mild irregularity of sustained junctional rhythm, may at times occur. This may result from a shift from one junctional pacemaker to another having a slightly different rate. In addition, at the onset of a run of junctional rhythm, a mild "warm-up" phenomenon may be observed; the rate increases slightly over the first several beats. Finally, junctional pacemakers located high in the junction may be subject to vagal influence; frank junctional arrhythmia may occur.

During junctional rhythm or AJR, the P-wave activity on the ECG may include the following:

1. Retrograde-P-waves precede each QRS by 0.12 sec. or less; or, retrograde-P-waves follow each QRS by up to about 0.40 sec. The P–R or R–P interval, respectively, is constant. (The underlying sinus rate is less than the retrograde-P-to-P rate.)
2. No P-waves are visible; the baseline is smooth. Either the underlying rhythm is AF, or retrograde-P-waves are buried in the QRSs (in which case, the underlying sinus rate is slower than the R–R rate).
3. Retrograde-P-waves are present with a repetitively changing relationship to the QRS-complexes, representing V–A Wenckebach periods, during which the R–P intervals progressively increase until either a dropped beat (no retrograde-P) or ventricular echo (early supraventricular QRS) occurs. Although V–A Wenckebach patterns may be apparent, one must carefully measure the retrograde-P-to-P intervals; if they are *constant*, one may really be dealing with an ectopic (low) atrial pacemaker dissociated from the junctional-QRSs (an early QRS, if it occurs, then becomes an antegrade capture by the ectopic atrial focus, rather than a ventricular echo).
4. Sinus, atrial flutter waves, or nonretrograde ectopic P-waves (ectopic atrial rhythm or NPAT) are present, and are dissociated from the junctional-QRSs. Early supraventricular QRSs are likely to be antegrade captures.

In digitalis excess, the junctional rate is proportional to the degree of toxicity. The rate accelerates or decelerates *slowly* (over days). In AJR due to acute myocardial infarction, cardiac trauma or surgery, or catecholamine administration, *the heart rate may accelerate over several hours.* In *most, but not all cases* of digitalis toxicity, AJR is accompanied by some degree of heart block.

Junctional rhythm and AJR are *perfectly regular.* Irregularities in the rhythm may be due to:

1. Early beats (antegrade captures, ventricular echoes, PJCs). These early QRSs may have functional aberration.
2. Sudden "pauses" caused by resetting of the junction by concealed conduction from a sinus-P or by an abortive ventricular echo (the junctional impulse reaches the upper A–V node, bounces down the other dual pathway, reaches the junction and resets the junctional pacemaker, but does not reach the ventricle). This will be discussed in Section IV.
3. Transient slowing of the junctional pacemaker, occurring spontaneously or induced by a capture or ventricular echo (see ECG IV–15). This type of *transient junctional pacemaker depression* is rare, occurring in digitalis-toxic patients with severe heart disease.
4. Transient increase in the heart rate, by one or more early QRSs precisely doubling the heart rate or by several early QRSs in a cluster, with a "group-beating"* pattern and no evidence they are captures or ventricular echoes. This implies that the true junctional rate is *double* the apparent rate (with 2:1 junctional-ventricular block being present). The increase in rate represents a transient return to 1:1 or Wenckebach conduction.
5. Consistent "group beating," where the R–R intervals progressively decrease, followed by a pause; this pattern is *repetitive,* resulting in a *regularly irregular* rhythm. There is advanced digitalis toxicity, with junctional-ventricular block of Wenckebach type.
6. Junctional arrhythmia, occasionally seen in young, healthy individuals having heightened vagal tone. In such cases there is significant concomitant sinus arrhythmia with occasional captures (i.e., incomplete A–V dissociation); both sinus and junction speed up and slow together. During the speed-up phases, the junctional rate may exceed 60 bpm; this is without significance (see ECG IV–14).

In junctional rhythm or AJR, the R–R interval between two consecutive junctional beats is measured to determine the junctional rate. If a premature ventricular beat (PVC) or early supraventricular beat (antegrade capture or ventricular echo) occurs, measuring *back one junctional cycle* from the beginning of the subsequent junctional beat permits determination of the point at which the PVC or early beat reset the junctional pacemaker. This usually occurs around the *end* of the PVC, since the ventricular impulse must conduct retrogradely to the junction. In the case of antegrade captures or ventricular echoes, the reset point is at or slightly prior to the *beginning* of the early beat, since the preceding P-wave traverses the junctional area before reaching the ventricle. The R–R interval between a capture/echo and subsequent junctional beat may therefore be either the same as or slightly less than* the R–R between two consecutive junctional beats.

Occasionally, junctional rhythm with PVCs in bigeminy** occurs. Since no two consecutive junctional beats occur, the true junctional rate cannot be ascertained. It may range from the apparent junctional rate to twice the apparent rate, depending on the presence and extent of concealed retrograde conduction from the PVC. This is illustrated in Figure I–4. If there is virtually no retrograde conduction, the true and apparent junctional rates are one and the same. If there is retrograde conduction which does not reach the junction, but which renders the distal conducting system refractory, the true junctional rate *could be double* the apparent rate; every other impulse fails to conduct. If the retrograde impulse from the PVC reaches and resets the junction, the true junctional rate is intermediate between the apparent rate and double the apparent rate. The exact rate cannot be determined, since it depends on the point of reset of the junction by the retrograde impulse.

Finally, it must be remembered that the "junctional beats" seen on the ECG really represent the antegrade capture of the ventricles by the junctional impulse; the retrograde-P-waves represent retrograde atrial capture. The actual junctional discharge cannot be seen on the surface ECG,*** just as the actual sinus discharge cannot be seen (sinus-P-waves represent the *atrial activation* by the sinus impulse). Keeping this in mind permits the understanding of the concepts of (1) a true junctional rate faster than the apparent rate, and (2) junctional-ventricular Wenckebach conduction, during the pause of which one junctional impulse fails to conduct.

Junctional Rhythm in AF

As previously discussed, regularization of the heart rate in AF indicates complete A–V nodal block and junctional rhythm. The cause is almost

---

*The R–R intervals progressively decrease, followed by a pause equal to less than the sum of the previous two R–R intervals, suggesting some type of Wenckebach period.

---

*If the junction to QRS interval (i.e., the "H–V" interval, as measured on the bundle of His electrogram) of the capture/echo is *slightly longer* than that of the junctional beat, then the R–R interval between the capture/echo and junctional beat is *slightly less* than that between two junctional beats.
**That is, each junctional beat is followed by a PVC.
***It can be seen in a special intracardiac recording of the His bundle electrogram. Promising new techniques may permit the routine recording of the His bundle on the surface electrocardiogram.

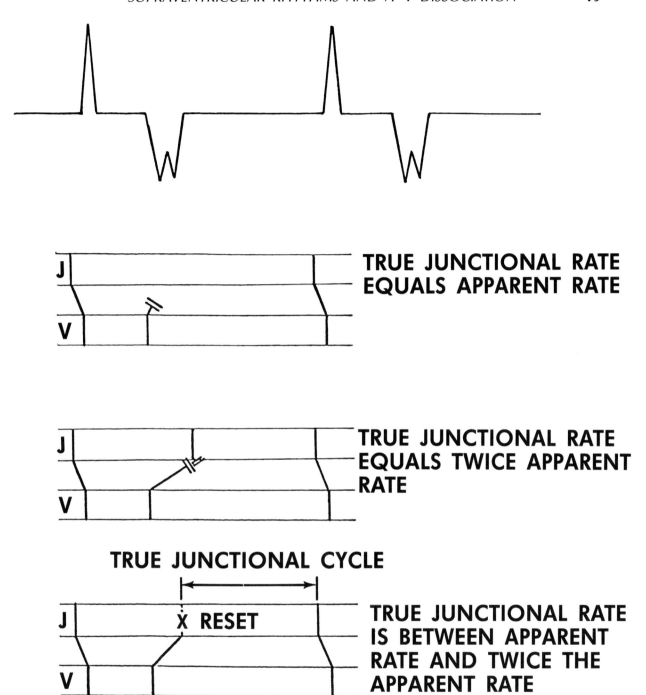

TRUE JUNCTIONAL RATE EQUALS APPARENT RATE

TRUE JUNCTIONAL RATE EQUALS TWICE APPARENT RATE

TRUE JUNCTIONAL CYCLE

Ẋ RESET

TRUE JUNCTIONAL RATE IS BETWEEN APPARENT RATE AND TWICE THE APPARENT RATE

Figure I–4. Junctional rhythm with PVCs in bigeminy.

invariably digitalis toxicity. As the digitalis level increases in AF, the ventricular response decreases; as advanced A–V nodal block develops, increasingly lengthy periods of regularity, representing periods of junctional escape rhythm, ensue. The rhythm finally becomes perfectly regular; the A–V nodal block is now complete. With further increase of the digitalis level, the junctional

rate progressively accelerates. At some point, usually at rates above 120 bpm, a *second level* of block, in the His-Purkinje system, develops. This junctional-ventricular block is of Wenckebach type. The heart rate is *regularly irregular,* with repetitive "group beating" (e.g., 4:3 periods appear as repetitive clusters of three beats followed by a pause; the R–R intervals progressively *decrease* before the pause).* This *regularly irregular* rhythm must never be confused with the *irregularly irregular* rhythm of ordinary AF.

Summary

The following diagnostic approach to all rhythms, both supraventricular and, as we shall later discuss, ventricular, should be used: Identify the P-waves. What is the atrial rate and morphol-

ogy? Identify the QRS-complexes. What is the relationship between the two? If there are periods of A–V dissociation, what is the junctional escape rate (i.e., normal or accelerated)? Is heart block present (i.e., P-waves that are in a position to capture, but do not)?* Finally, in cases of junctional rhythm with early beats, are the early beats sinus captures or ventricular echoes? In either case, what is the underlying sinus rate? Is the rhythm *regularly irregular*, with "group beating" indicative of Wenckebach periods? A methodical, step-by-step approach, utilizing long rhythm strips, multiple leads, and, if necessary, vagal maneuvers, almost always yields the correct diagnosis.

---

*In atrial flutter or NPAT, complete A–V nodal block and AJR with junctional-ventricular Wenckebach periods can be differentiated from simple A–V (nodal) Wenckebach periods. In simple A–V Wenckebach periods, all homologous QRSs (i.e., all the first QRSs of each comparable group, all the second QRSs, etc.) have the same P–R intervals; in addition, the P–R intervals progressively increase. In complete A–V nodal block and AJR with junctional-ventricular Wenckebach periods, there is complete A–V dissociation.

---

*As we shall see in Section II, in cases of advanced heart block, the presence of at least two consecutively conducted P-waves is necessary to identify the site of block.

SECTION I
Electrocardiograms

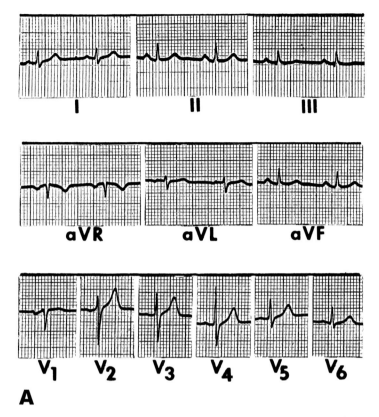

A

ECG I–1.   A. *Normal sinus rhythm.* The P-waves have sinus morphology. Each P-wave is followed by a QRS; each QRS is preceded by a P-wave. Additional examples of normal sinus rhythm are seen in the next four electrocardiograms (B through E).

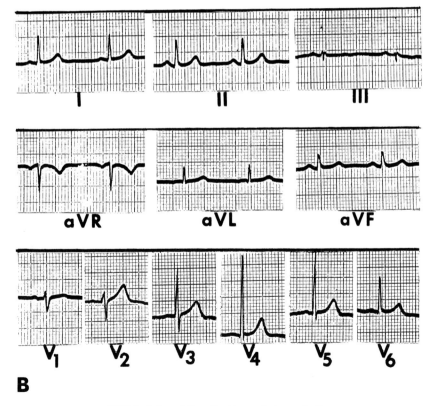

B

ECG I–1 (cont'd).   B. *Normal sinus rhythm.*

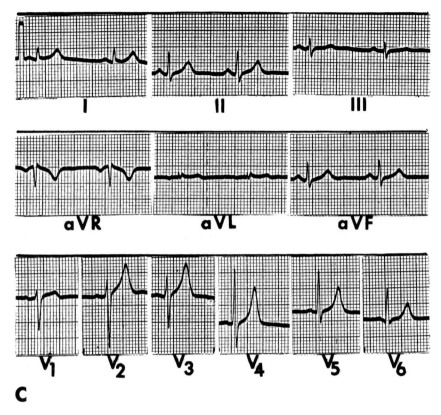

ECG I–1 (cont'd).   C. *Normal sinus rhythm.*

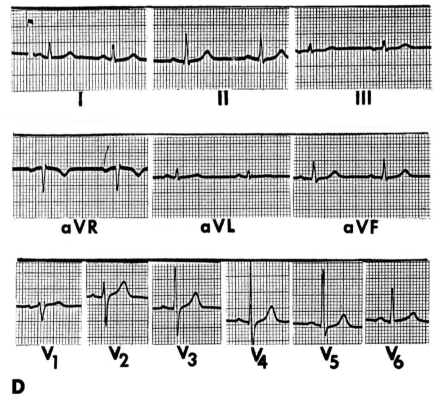

ECG I–1 (cont'd).   D. *Normal sinus rhythm.*

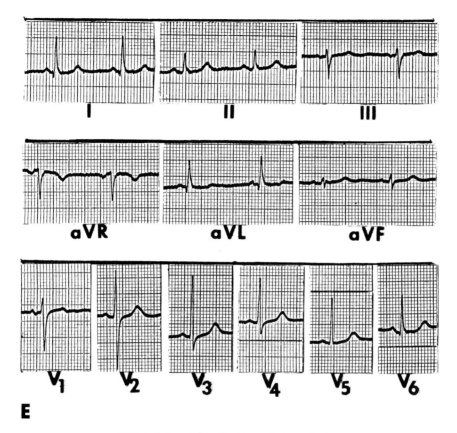

ECG I–1 (cont'd). E. *Normal sinus rhythm.*

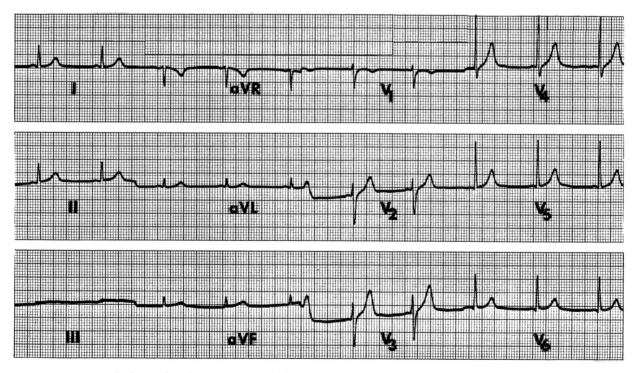

ECG I–2. *Sinus rhythm with a short P–R interval.* The P-waves have sinus morphology, but the P–R interval is only 0.10 second. The QRS-complexes do not show initial slurring, excluding the Wolff-Parkinson-White (W-P-W) syndrome. The short P–R interval may be caused by a heightened adrenergic state or an A–V nodal bypass tract (i.e., James bundle, the Lown-Ganong-Levine syndrome).

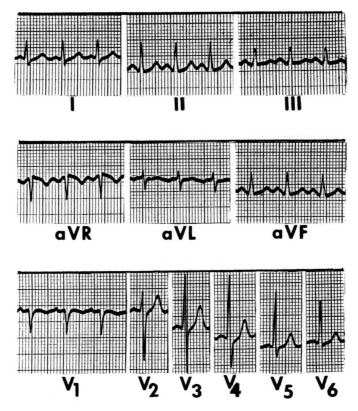

ECG I–3. *Sinus tachycardia.* The heart rate is 130 bpm.

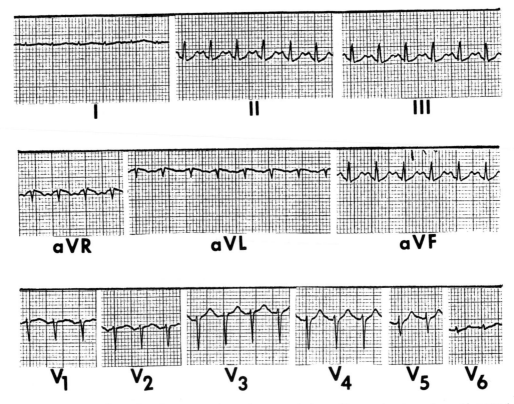

ECG I–4. *Marked sinus tachycardia.* The P-waves have sinus morphology. The rate is extremely rapid at 188 bpm. Such a rapid rate could only be found in a younger adult. In fact, the patient was a 26-year-old burn patient with sepsis.

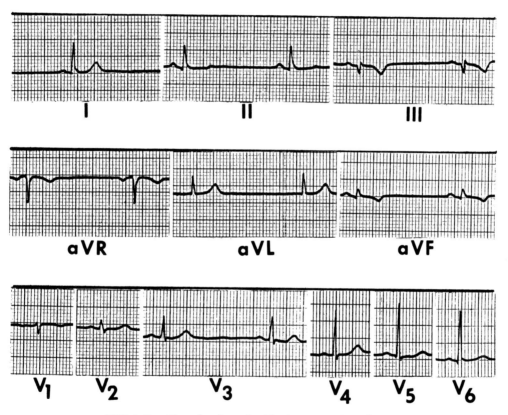

ECG I–5. *Sinus bradycardia.* The heart rate is 47 bpm.

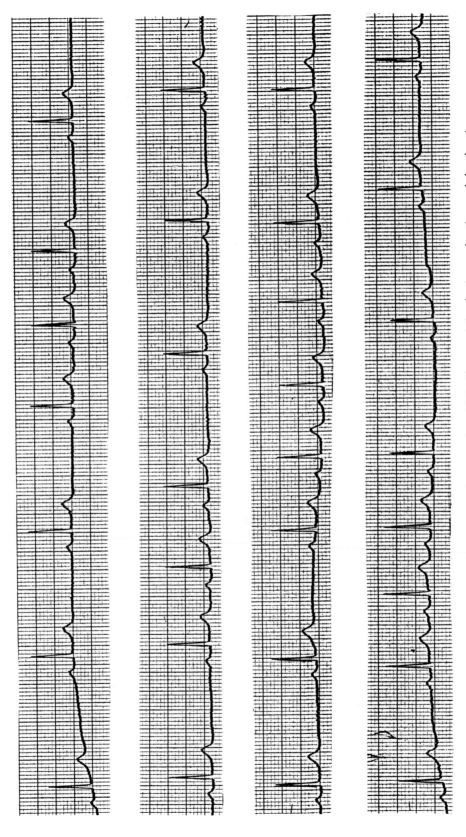

ECG I-6. *Sinus arrhythmia.* The heart rate varies by more than 10%. Characteristic phasic acceleration and deceleration are seen.

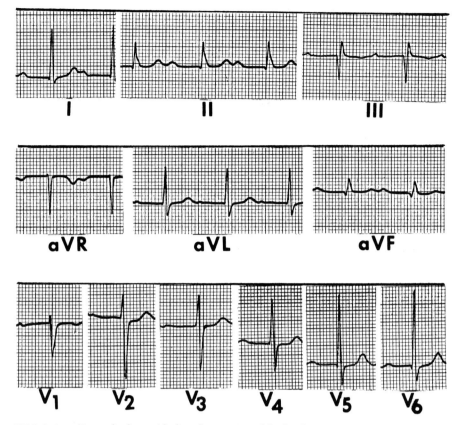

ECG I–7. *Sinus rhythm with first-degree A–V block.* The P–R interval is 0.38 sec.

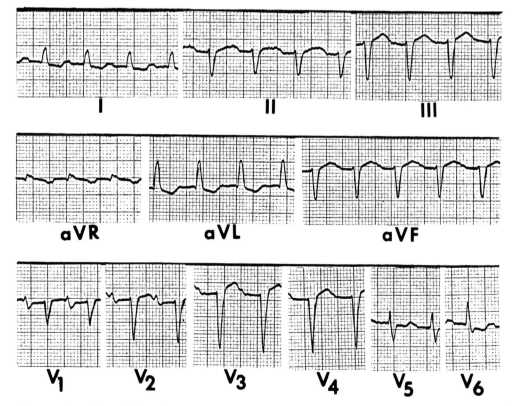

ECG I–8. *Sinus tachycardia with first-degree A–V block.* The P-waves are partially buried in the preceding T-waves and are best seen in Leads V_1 and V_2.

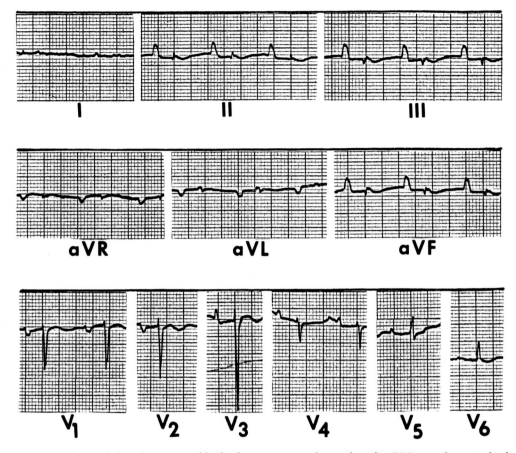

I   II   III

aVR   aVL   aVF

V_1 V_2 V_3 V_4 V_5 V_6

ECG I–9. *Sinus rhythm with first-degree A–V block.* The P-waves are larger than the QRS-complexes in the frontal leads. Perusal of Lead II alone might easily result in an erroneous diagnosis.

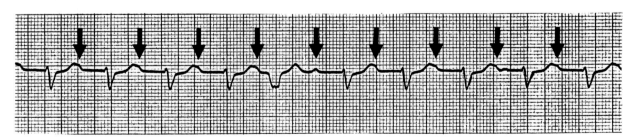

ECG I–10. *Sinus rhythm with first-degree A–V block.* Note the slight deformity of the T-waves, suggesting a buried P-wave in each (arrows). Following the PVC, a P-wave is unmasked. Note that the unmasked P-wave comes on time, indicating there are indeed P-waves buried in the Ts.

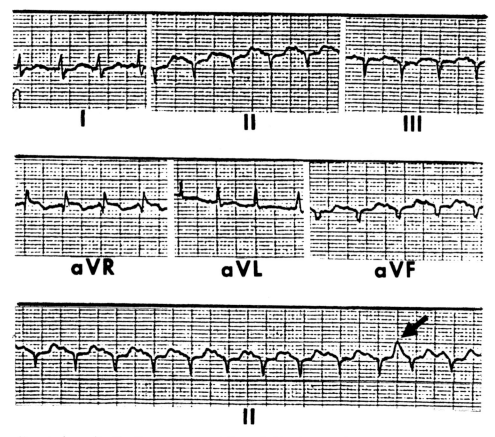

ECG I–11. *Sinus tachycardia.* The P-waves are partially buried in the preceding T-waves and have sinus morphology. Although the heart rate is 150 bpm, slight irregularity is present. This slight irregularity, as well as the presence of a PAC (arrow), indicates sinus tachycardia rather than PAT.

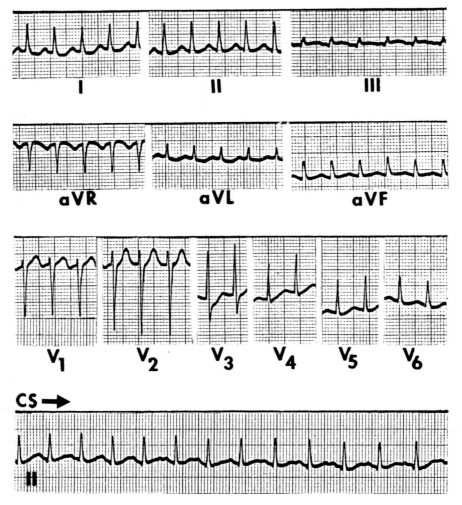

ECG I–12. *Sinus tachycardia.* Inspection reveals a supraventricular tachycardia at 167 bpm. P-waves are not apparent, although the slight negative deflections (arrow) immediately following the T-waves in V₁ are suspicious. Carotid sinus (CS) massage slightly slows the rate, causing the sinus-P-waves to separate from the Ts.

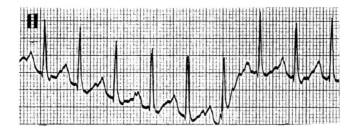

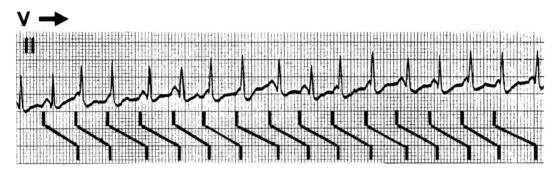

ECG I–13. *Sinus tachycardia with marked, varying first-degree A–V block.* In the control ECG, sinus tachycardia is present. The P-waves sit atop the Ts. Following a vagal (V) surge induced by Tensilon, marked, varying first-degree A–V block is produced. This results in the interesting situation in which a P-wave conducts to produce the QRS *after* the one which immediately follows it. Post-Tensilon, the P-wave rate remains constant (at 150 bpm). The P–R intervals vary from 0.44 to 0.50 sec. The R–R intervals vary because of the varying P–R intervals. This R–R variation excludes the diagnosis of complete A–V dissociation with a markedly accelerated junctional rhythm.

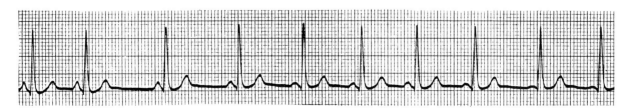

ECG I–14. *Wandering atrial pacemaker.* The atrial rate and morphology vary.

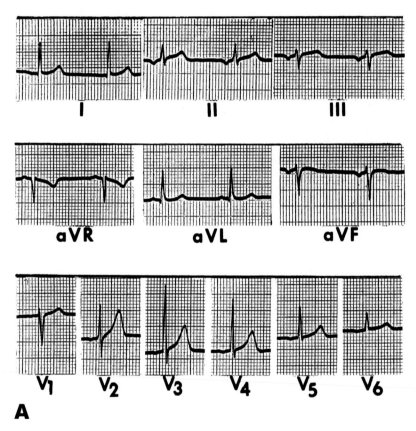

ECG I–15. *Ectopic atrial rhythm.* The P-waves do not have sinus morphology. The P–R intervals are at least 0.12 sec. A. Ectopic atrial rhythm ("coronary sinus rhythm").

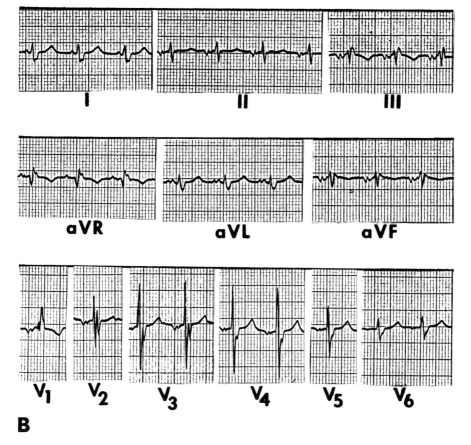

ECG I–15 (cont'd).   B. Ectopic atrial rhythm/tachycardia.

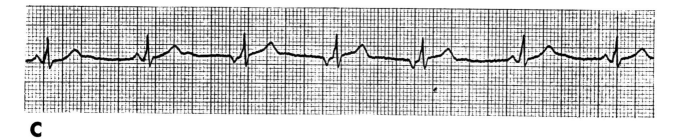

ECG I–15 (cont'd).   C. Rhythm varies between sinus and ectopic atrial rhythm.

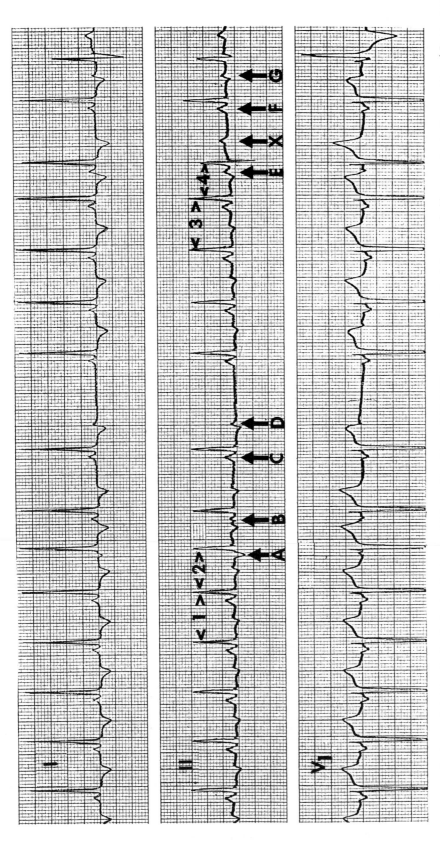

ECG I-16. *Sinus rhythm with PACs.* The basic rhythm is sinus at 98 bpm. The 6th and 7th QRSs are premature. Each is preceded by an ectopic P-wave (A and B, respectively). Note that the two PACs arise from different atrial foci. Following the second PAC, there is another sinus beat. Note that the sinus-P-wave of this beat (C) follows the PAC by one sinus-cycle plus about 0.16 sec. During this increment of time, the PAC is in the process of entering the S–A node and resetting the sinus. Following this sinus beat there is an unexpected pause. Examination of the T-wave contained within the pause reveals a non-conducted PAC (D), which produces a deformity. Four additional sinus beats follow, after which there occurs a PAC (E), this time conducted with functional aberration of left anterior hemiblock type (note the left axis deviation). The functional aberration presumably occurs for E rather than for A or B because E is preceded by a more favorable "long-short" R–R cycle ratio. That is, in comparing A and E, the preceding long cycles are equal (1 = 3), but the short cycle immediately preceding E is shorter than that preceding A (4 < 2). Furthermore, D is non-conducted because it occurs even earlier. Coming at the tail-end of the preceding T-wave, it encounters a refractory A–V node and/or His-Purkinje system. Following E, there is another deflection (X). This represents a change in T-wave morphology, rather than another PAC. If it had been a PAC, the next sinus beat (F) would have appeared after an interval equal to one sinus-cycle plus an increment of 0.10 to 0.20 sec. (unless S–A node entrance block, whose spontaneous occurrence is extremely rare, had been present). In other words, the interval between X and F should have been approximately equal to that between B and C, if X had been a PAC. Since, for all practical purposes, S–A node entrance block can be discounted, sinus beat F appears too early to have been reset by X. The abnormal T-wave, represented by X, is secondary to the abnormal QRS caused by the functional aberration (i.e., abnormal depolarization results in abnormal repolarization). Following F, there is another PAC (G), this time conducted with functional aberration of RBBB type.

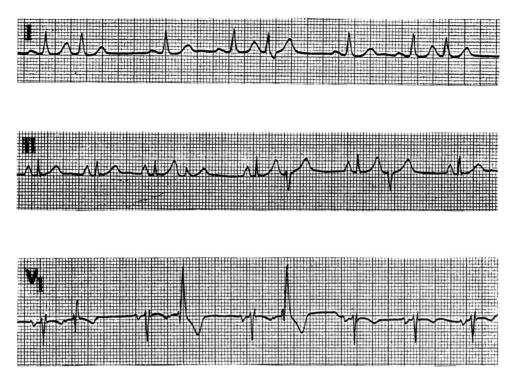

ECG I–17. *Sinus rhythm with PACs.* The extrasystoles are preceded by T-waves which are different from those not preceding the extrasystoles—taller in Lead II, notched in V₁. A number of the PACs are conducted with functional aberration, particularly during periods of atrial bigeminy. Can you tell why?

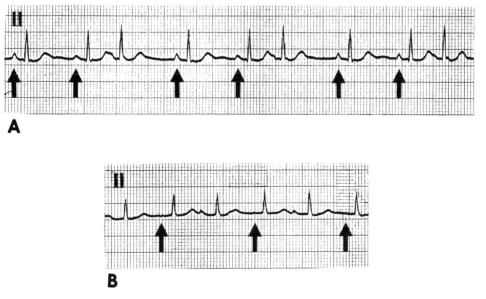

ECG I–18. *Ectopic atrial rhythm with PACs.* A. Wandering atrial pacemaker with PACs in trigeminy. The P-wave morphology of the dominant rhythm varies (arrows). B. Ectopic atrial rhythm with PACs in bigeminy. The P-wave morphology of the dominant rhythm is non-sinus (arrows). The PACs are conducted with first-degree A–V block because they are relatively early—coming at the end of the preceding T-waves, they encounter a still partially refractory A–V node.

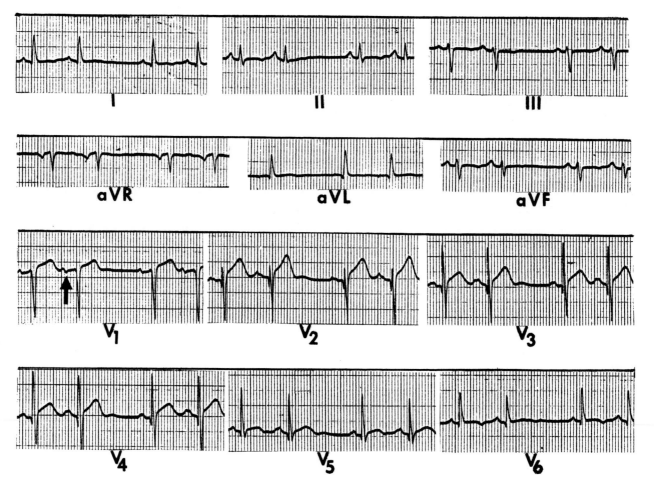

ECG I–19. *Sinus rhythm with perisinal PACs in bigeminy.* The PACs arise from a site close to the S–A node; hence, the ectopic P-waves are almost identical to those of the sinus. Careful inspection reveals the ectopic P-waves to be slightly larger in Leads II, aVR, aVF, and V_2, in addition to having a slightly deeper negative component (arrow) in Lead V_1. Nevertheless, the differences are certainly subtle. If no such differences had been detectable, the differential diagnosis would have been between sinus rhythm with perisinal PACs in bigeminy, and sinus tachycardia with 3:2 S–A Wenckebach periods.

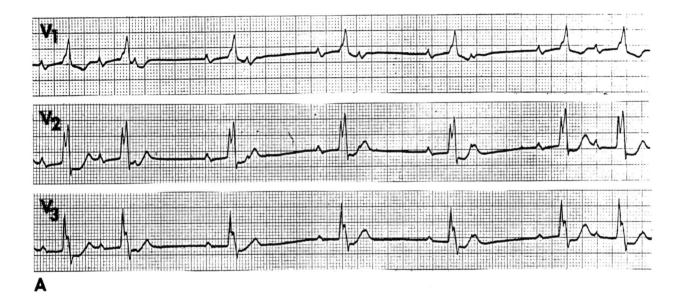

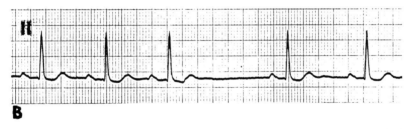

ECG I–20. *Non-conducted PACs.* Can you spot the ectopic P-waves? A. First-degree A–V block and RBBB are present. B. First-degree A–V block and sinus arrhythmia are present.

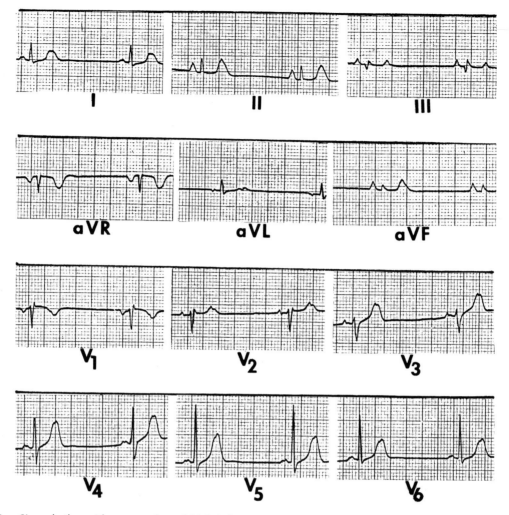

ECG I–21. *Sinus rhythm with non-conducted PACs in bigeminy.* Although all the T-waves are uniform, note their deformity—pointy and/or notched in the various leads. Pure T-waves never look like this.

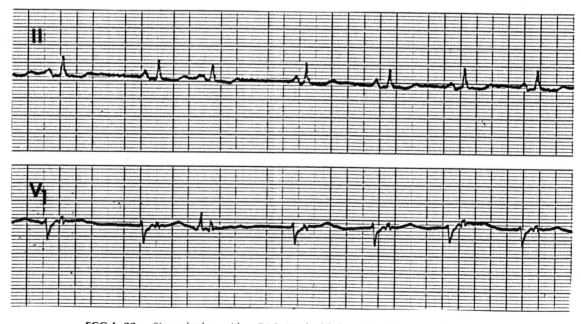

ECG I–22. *Sinus rhythm with a PAC.* Marked left atrial enlargement is present.

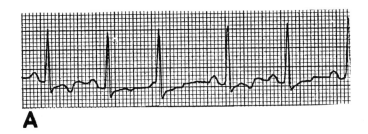

A

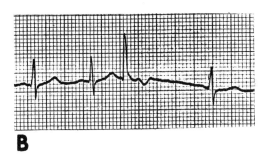

B

ECG I–23.   *PJCs.* A. The premature supraventricular beat sits atop a normally occurring sinus-P-wave. B. The premature supraventricular beat precedes a normally occurring sinus-P-wave. The PJC is slightly aberrant, either because of functional aberration or because it arises in one of the proximal bundle fascicles (i.e., is a premature subjunctional beat).

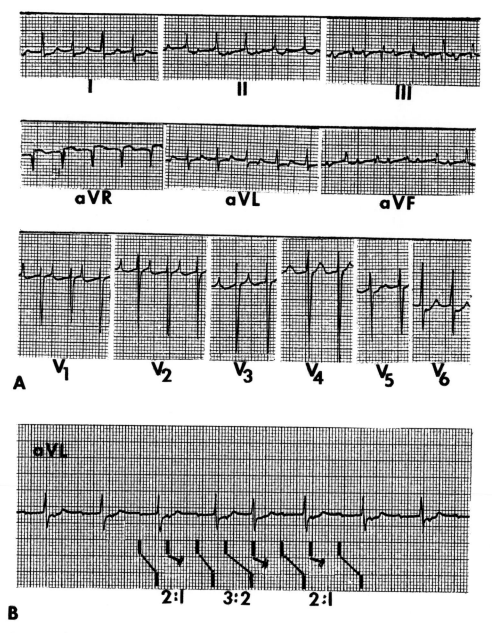

ECG I–24. *Paroxysmal ectopic atrial tachycardia (PAT).* A. The heart rate is 160 bpm and regular. The P-waves are non-sinus in morphology. First-degree A–V block is present. B. After propranolol, PAT is still present, but A–V conduction has decreased to 2:1 (one 3:2 period is also present).

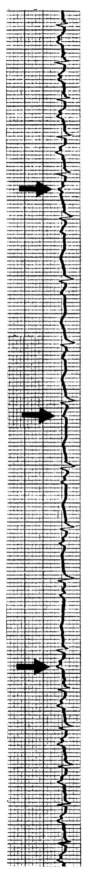

ECG I–25. *PAT.* Interestingly, following the termination of a run of PAT (first arrow), the ectopic pacemaker remains as the dominant escape rhythm for three beats. The sinus then emerges for four beats (second arrow). A PAC then triggers another run of PAT (third arrow).

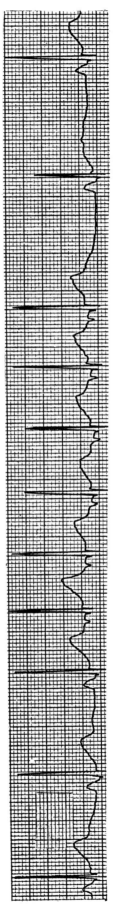

ECG I–26. *Sinus bradycardia with a run of slow PAT.* The ectopic atrial focus fires somewhat irregularly at a rate between 88 and 100 bpm.

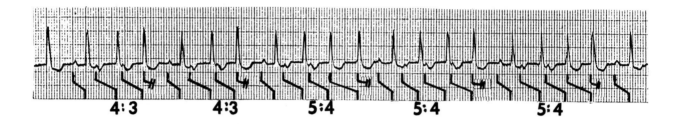

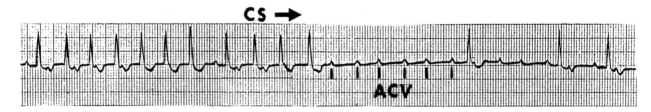

ECG I–27.   *PAT.* A–V conduction is close to 1:1 (the ratios of the various A–V Wenckebach periods are indicated). Following carotid massage (CS), A–V conduction transiently slows, revealing "long-short" atrial cycle variation (ACV). This variation is observed in some cases of both paroxysmal and nonparoxysmal atrial tachycardia. In this case, since A–V conduction approaches 1:1, the rhythm is PAT rather than digitalis-toxic "PAT with block" (NPAT). (Reproduced with permission from Childers, R., and Gambetta, M. Alternation of atrial cycle length in supraventricular tachycardia. J. Electrocardiol., *2*:213, 1978.)

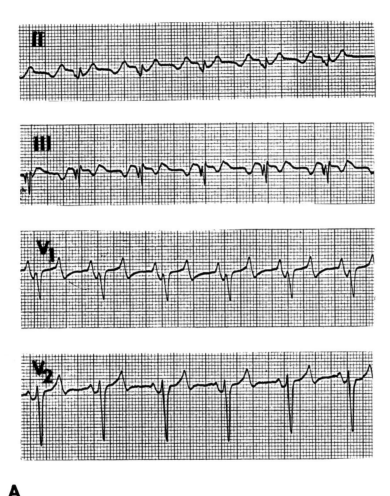

A

ECG I–28. *Nonparoxysmal atrial tachycardia (NPAT) with 2:1 A–V block.* Note that in some of the leads the second P-wave within the ST-T complex is less obvious. To avoid missing the diagnosis, multiple leads should be examined. In addition, when confronted with any ECG revealing "sinus rhythm" or "ectopic atrial rhythm" between 60 and 120 bpm, one should divide the obvious P–P interval in half and determine whether a deformity or deflection corresponding to a second P-wave is present at that point. Finally, note that, in all three cases, either of the two P-waves could have produced the QRS, since both P–R intervals fall between 0.12 and 0.60 sec. A. The atrial rate is 150 bpm.

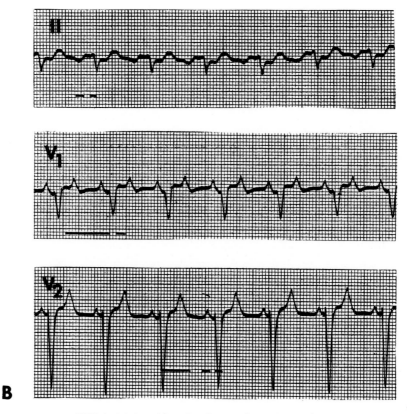

ECG I–28 (cont'd).   B. The atrial rate is 166 bpm.

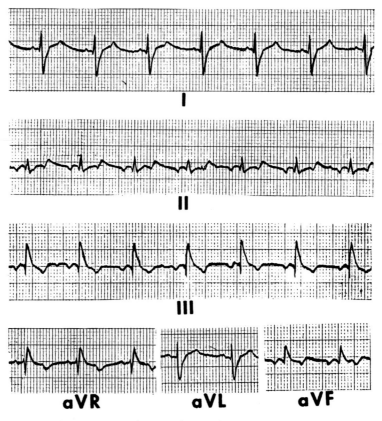

ECG I–28 (cont'd).   C. The atrial rate is 170 bpm.

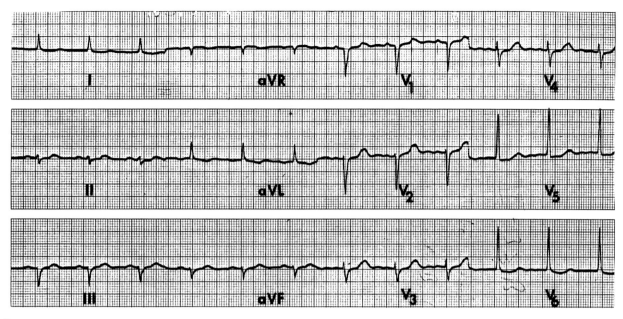

D

ECG I–28 (cont'd). D. The atrial rate is 144 bpm. The second P-wave slightly deforms the T-wave, particularly in Leads II, V_1, and V_2.

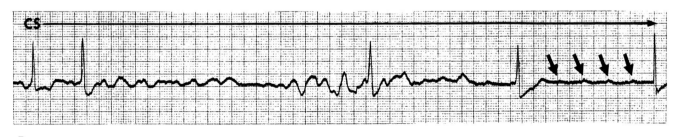

E

ECG I–28 (cont'd). E. (Same patient as I–28D) During carotid massage (CS), all the P-waves (arrows) are exposed.

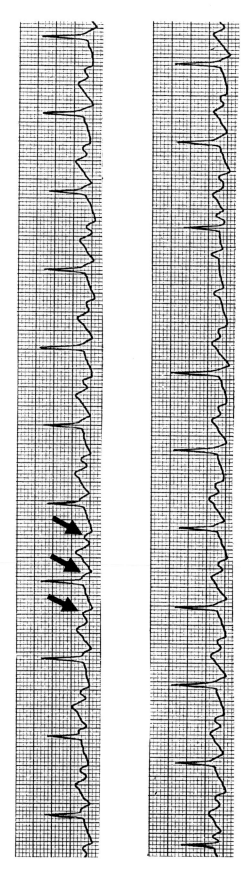

ECG I-29. *NPAT with 2:1 A–V block.* Top panel: dividing the obvious P–P interval in half reveals a second P-wave whose descending limb emerges from the QRS complex (arrows). Later (bottom panel), A–V conduction spontaneously decreases, revealing the true atrial rate (140 bpm).

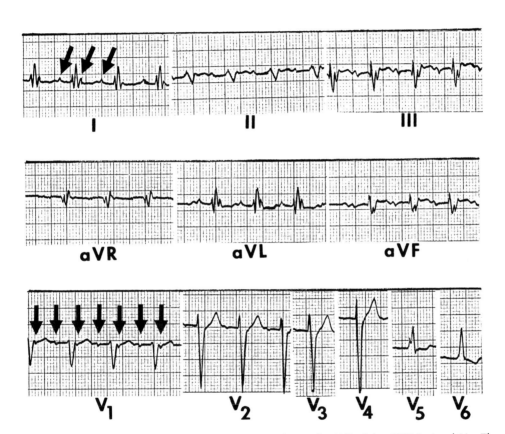

ECG I–30. *NPAT with 2:1 A–V block.* The second P-wave forms the "r" of the QRS in Lead V₁. The atrial rate is 214 bpm. Arrows point to P-waves. All the "V" leads are ½ standard.

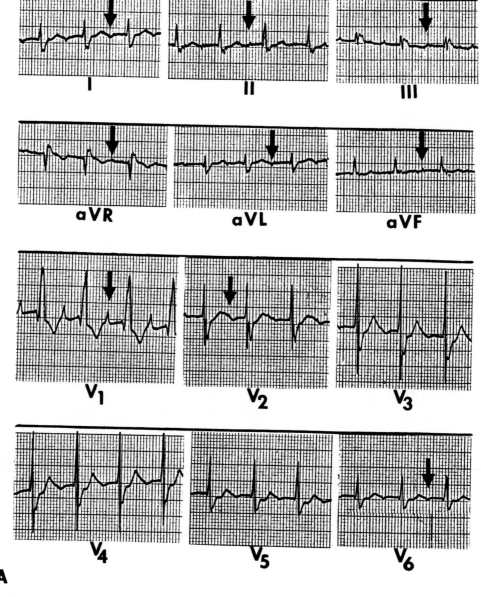

A

ECG I–31. *NPAT with 2:1 A–V block.* A. At first glance, the rhythm appears to be an ectopic atrial rhythm at a rate of 105 bpm. P-waves in a number of the leads are indicated by arrows. Please note that if the obvious P–P interval is divided in half, the second P-wave would fall in the middle of the QRS-complex, which is widened by RBBB, and would, therefore, be completely obscured. What can one do to try to unmask a possible second P-wave?

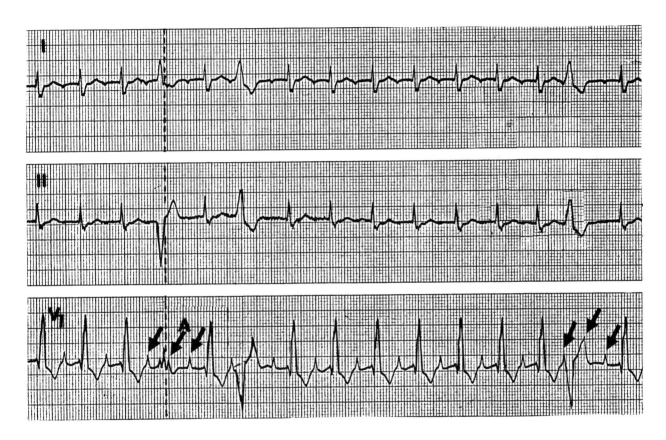

B

ECG I–31 (cont'd). B. Several PVCs spontaneously occur. Careful inspection of Lead V₁ at the time of the PVCs reveals the extra P-waves, which are unmasked. Note that the P-wave labeled A forms the third prong of a "crown," which is comprised of PVC (first two prongs) plus P-wave; this third prong occurs *beyond the end* of the PVC (broken line).

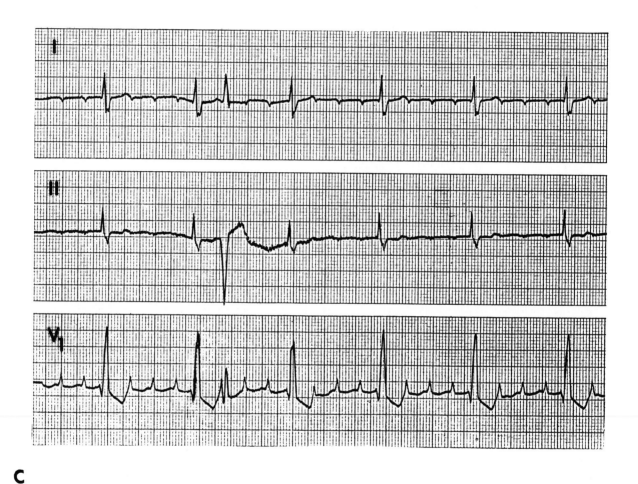

C

ECG I–31 (cont'd).   C. A few moments later, A–V conduction spontaneously decreased to 4:1, confirming the true atrial rate of 210 bpm. A PVC is also present.

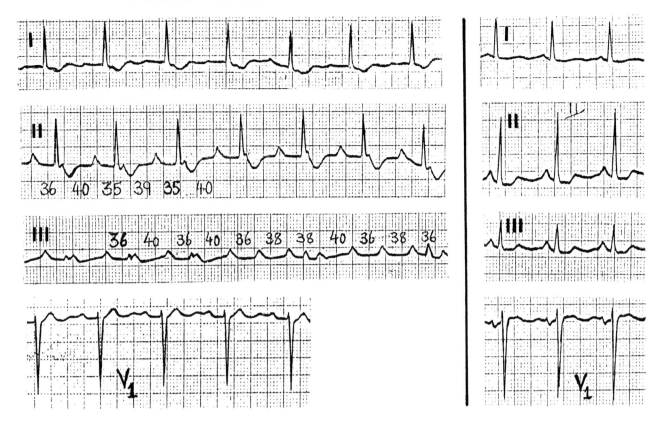

ECG I–32.   NPAT with 2:1 A–V block. This is shown in the ECG on the left. The second P-wave is partially buried in the QRS. The atrial rate varies between 150 and 170 bpm. "Long–short" atrial cycle variation, illustrated in Leads II and III, is present. Note the similarity of the ectopic P-waves in the ECG on the left to those of the sinus in the ECG on the right. That ECG represents the last tracing taken before the patient became digitalis-toxic. Superficial examination of the ECG on the left could easily lead to the erroneous conclusion that only first-degree A–V block had occurred. Note the transient increase in A–V block in Lead III. (Reproduced with permission from Childers, R., and Gambetta, M. Alternation of atrial cycle length in supraventricular tachycardia. J. Electrocardiol., *2*:213, 1978.)

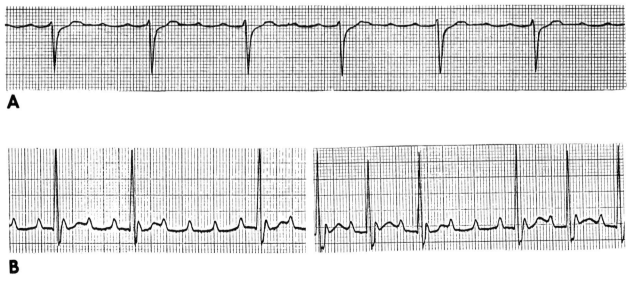

ECG I–33.   *NPAT with A–V block.* A. 4:1 A–V block. B. Variable A–V block. (Stein, E. *The Electrocardiogram: A Self-Study Course in Clinical Electrocardiography.* Courtesy of W. B. Saunders Co., 1976.)

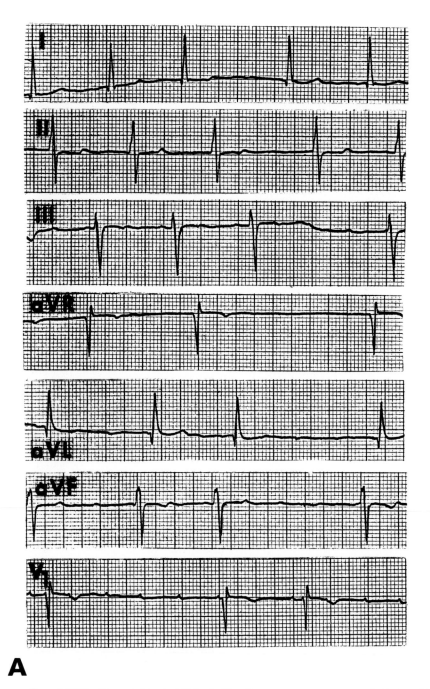

A

ECG I–34. A. *Low-voltage NPAT with variable A–V block.* The P-waves are apparent only in Lead V$_1$. The patient is extremely digitalis-toxic. The ECG could easily be mistaken for AF with a moderate response.

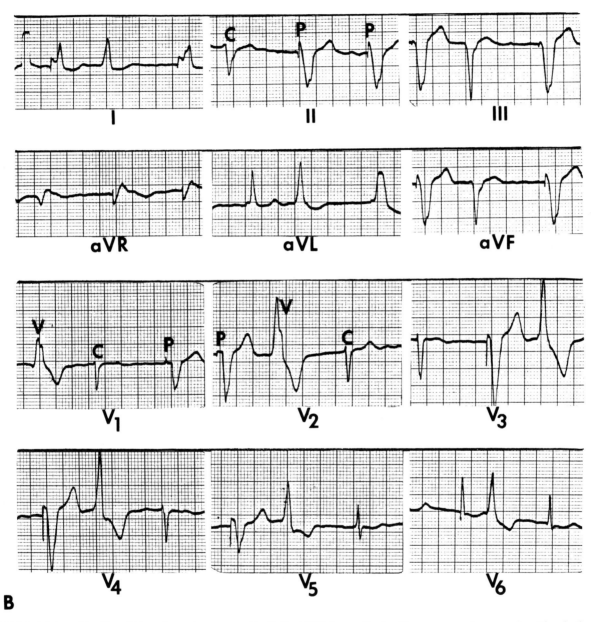

B

ECG I–34 (cont'd—B and C are from the same patient). B. *NPAT in a patient with a permanent pacemaker.* The rhythm is atrial fibrillation. Note the undulating baseline and the absence of discrete P-waves. There are supraventricular captures (C), paced beats (P), and PVCs (V).

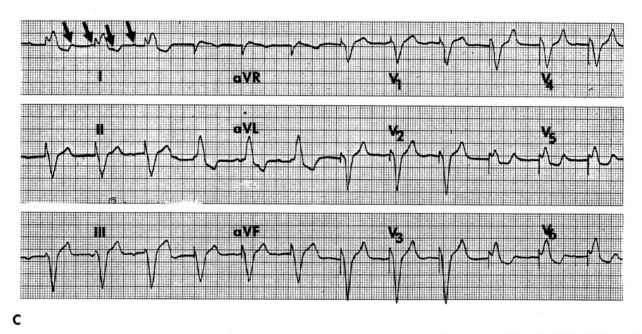

C

ECG I–34 (cont'd). C. *NPAT.* There are now discrete P-waves (arrows) in the baseline at a rate of 166 bpm. All the beats are paced, indicating there is now complete A–V block. In patients with permanent pacemakers, careful examination of the underlying atrial rhythm may be the only tipoff to the development of digitalis toxicity, and should always be performed.

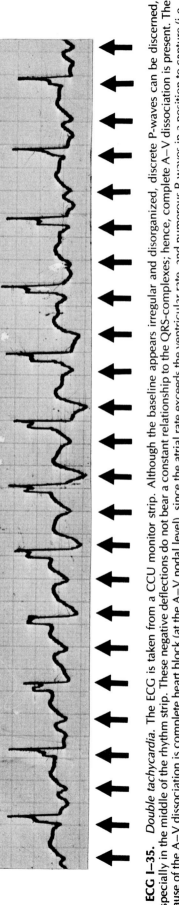

ECG I–35.   *Double tachycardia.* The ECG is taken from a CCU monitor strip. Although the baseline appears irregular and disorganized, discrete P-waves can be discerned, especially in the middle of the rhythm strip. These negative deflections do not bear a constant relationship to the QRS-complexes; hence, complete A–V dissociation is present. The cause of the A–V dissociation is complete heart block (at the A–V nodal level), since the atrial rate exceeds the ventricular rate, and numerous P-waves in a position to capture (i.e., produce early QRSs) fail to do so. Note the pseudo-Q and pseudo-S-waves formed by the merger of the negative P-waves with the QRSs. This rhythm represents NPAT (at 188 bpm) with complete A–V block and accelerated junctional rhythm (at 107 bpm). This so-called "double tachycardia" is indicative of advanced digitalis toxicity.

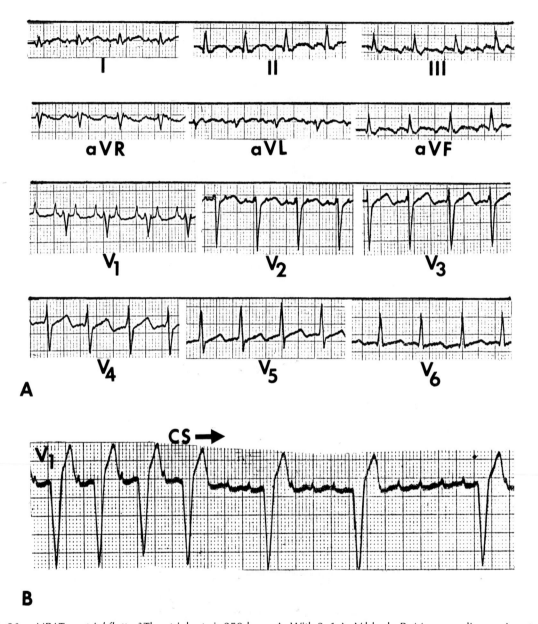

ECG I–36.   *NPAT or atrial flutter?* The atrial rate is 250 bpm. A. With 2:1 A–V block. B. Masquerading as sinus tachycardia with first-degree A–V block. LBBB is present. The extra P-waves are unmasked by carotid massage (CS).

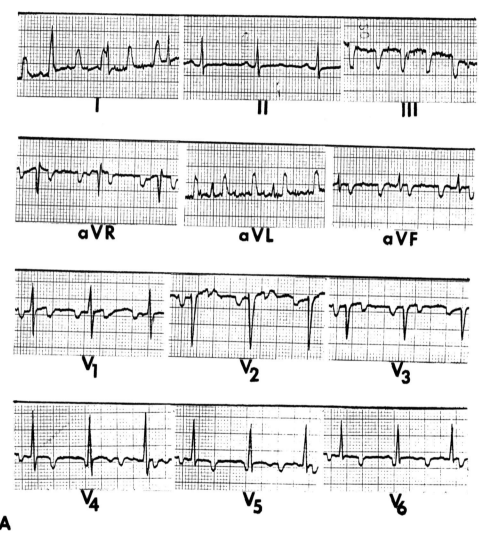

ECG I–37. *Artifactual NPAT with A–V block.* A. Note the gross irregularity of the "atrial rate" as well as, of course, the absence of artifact in Lead II.

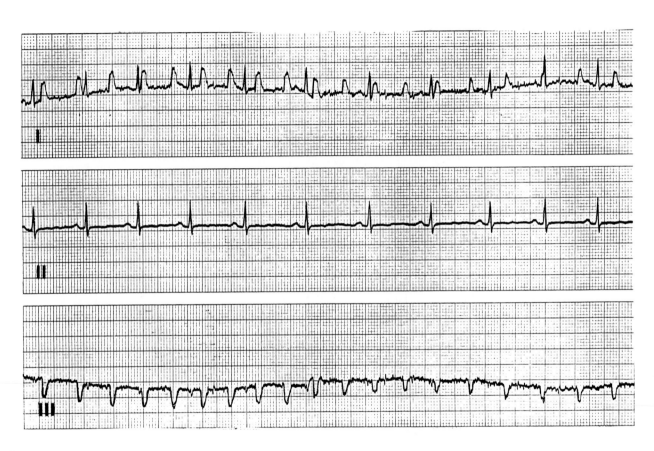

B

ECG I–37 (cont'd).   B. Note the absence of artifact in Lead II, which is simultaneous with Leads I and III.

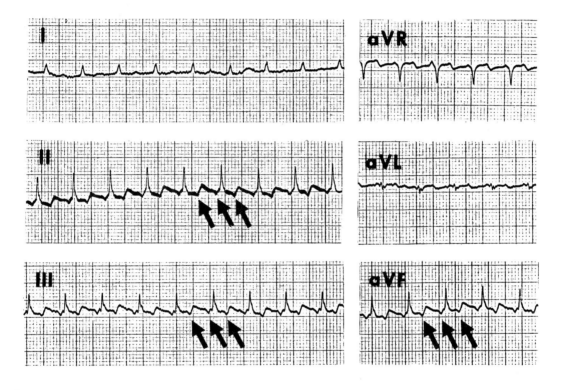

A

ECG I–38. *Atrial flutter.* In each case, note the angularity ("saw-tooth") of the flutter waves (arrows), which have uniform morphology and are perfectly regular at approximately 300 bpm. A. 2:1 A–V conduction.

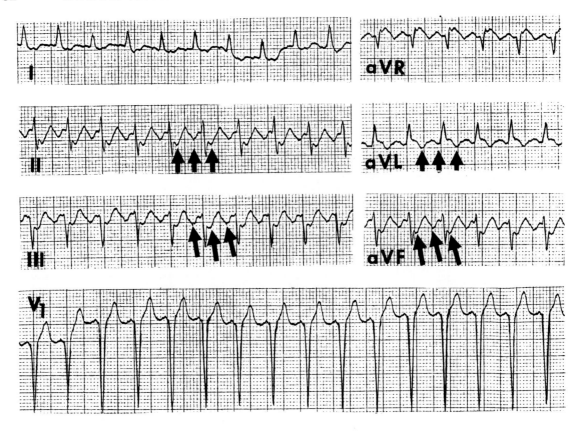

B

ECG I-38 (cont'd).   B. 2:1 A–V conduction. Note how Lead V₁ could be mistaken for sinus tachycardia.

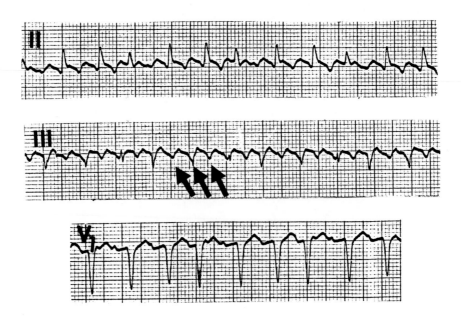

C

ECG I-38 (cont'd).   C. Variable rapid response. The "saw-tooth" flutter waves are best seen in Lead III.

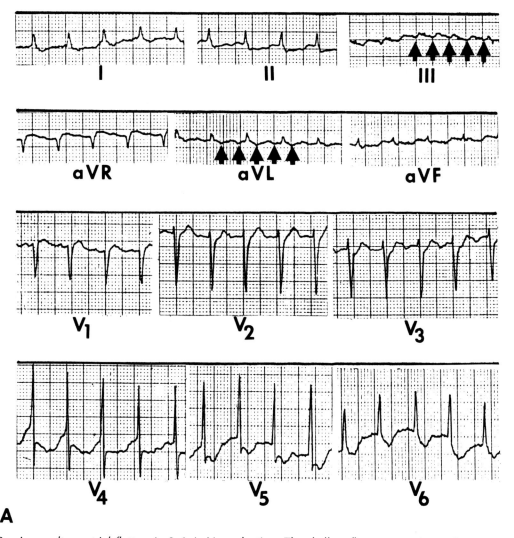

A

ECG I–39. *Low voltage atrial flutter.* A. 2:1 A–V conduction. The shallow flutter waves (arrows) are appreciated by careful inspection of Leads III and aVL. As in ECG I–38B, Lead V₁ could easily be mistaken for sinus tachycardia.

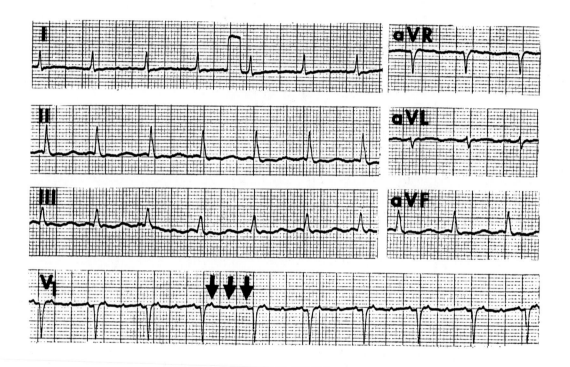

B

ECG I–39 (cont'd).   B. 3:1 A–V conduction. Discrete flutter waves are seen only in Lead V$_1$. The 3:1 A–V conducting ratio is unusual, and actually represents bilevel block within the A–V node (see Section II).

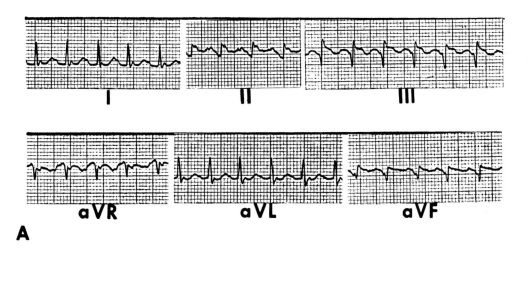

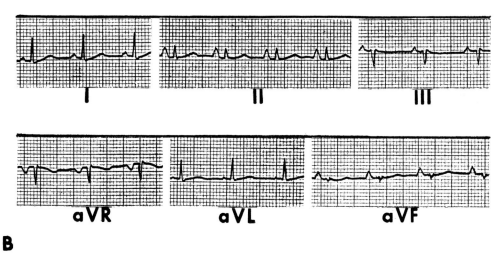

ECG I–40. A. Atrial flutter with 2:1 A–V conduction. The juxtaposition of the relatively large, angular flutter waves with the relatively small QRS-complexes produces the illusion of an acute inferior wall myocardial infarction. B. After conversion to sinus rhythm the wide pseudo-Q-waves and pseudo-ST-elevation are no longer present.

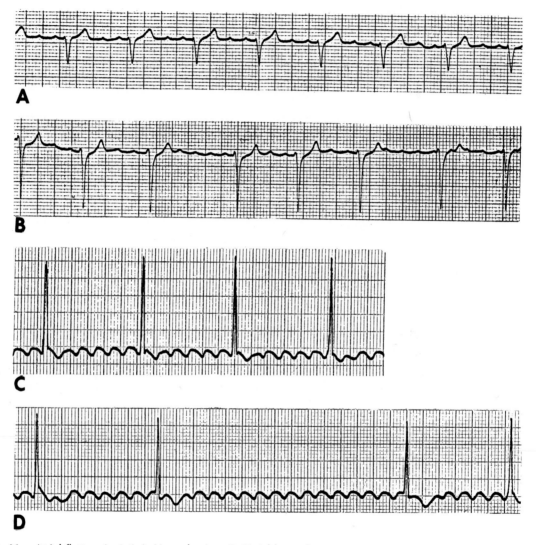

ECG I–41.   Atrial flutter. A. 4:1 A–V conduction. B. Variable moderate response. C. 6:1 A–V conduction. D. Variable slow response. High grade A–V block is present. (C and D. Stein, E. *The Electrocardiogram: A Self-Study Course in Clinical Electrocardiography.* Courtesy of W. B. Saunders Co., 1976.)

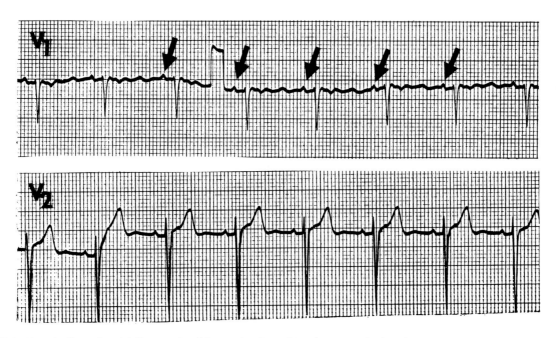

ECG I–42. Artifactual atrial flutter. Careful examination of Lead V₁ reveals that the true sinus-P-waves (arrows) look different than the other undulations. In Lead V₂ the artifact has disappeared.

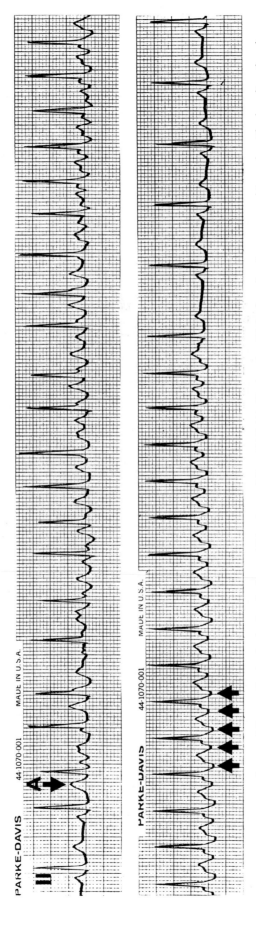

ECG 1–43. *Paroxysmal AF and flutter.* The basic rhythm is sinus. AF is triggered by a PAC (A). During the AF the baseline is coarse and irregular. The baseline then becomes regular and uniform; the rhythm has become atrial flutter. This is well seen in the second panel where the series of arrows point to some of the flutter waves. The flutter then self-terminates, and sinus rhythm resumes. During the AF, the ventricular response is rapid, averaging 150 bpm. During the atrial flutter, A–V conduction is 2:1, with the resulting heart rate also 150 bpm. This is a long Lead II.

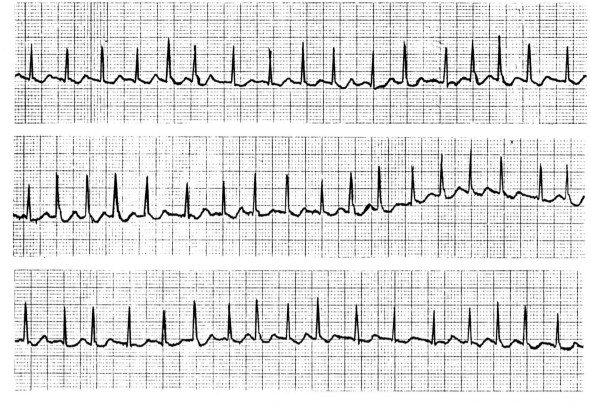

ECG I–44. *AF with a rapid ventricular response.* The heart rate is approximately 160 bpm. The baseline is irregular and no discrete P-waves are seen.

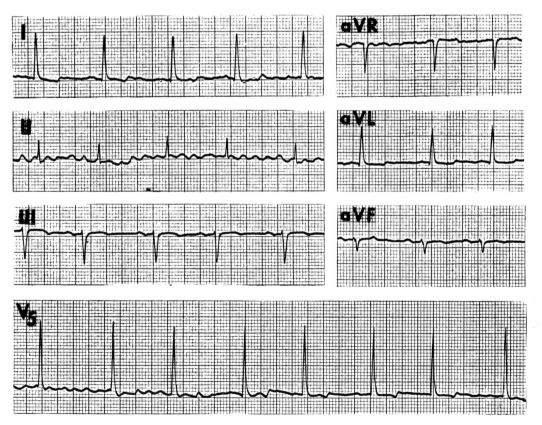

ECG I–45. *AF with a moderate ventricular response.* The heart rate is 70–80 bpm. In some of the leads the baseline is coarse, but the undulations are irregular and nonuniform, excluding atrial flutter.

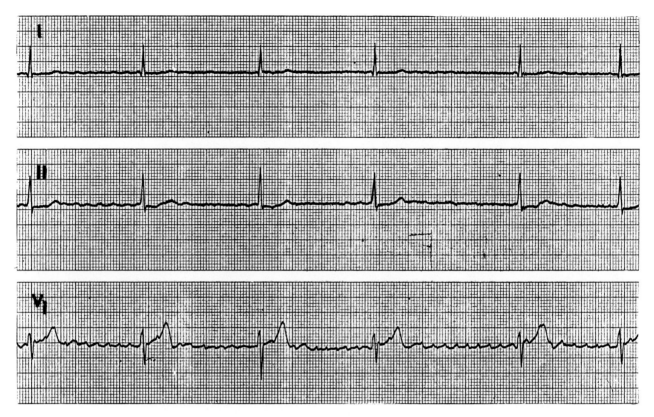

ECG I–46. *AF with a slow ventricular response.* The heart rate is approximately 40 bpm. The baseline undulations in Lead V₁ are irregular and non-uniform. The three leads are simultaneous.

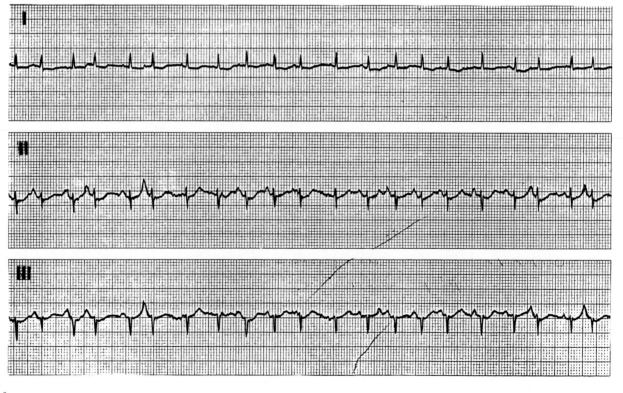

A

ECG I–47. A. *Chaotic atrial tachycardia.* The rhythm is rapid and irregular, but discrete P-waves of varying rate and morphology are present. Electrocardiograms B and C are additional examples of chaotic atrial tachycardia.

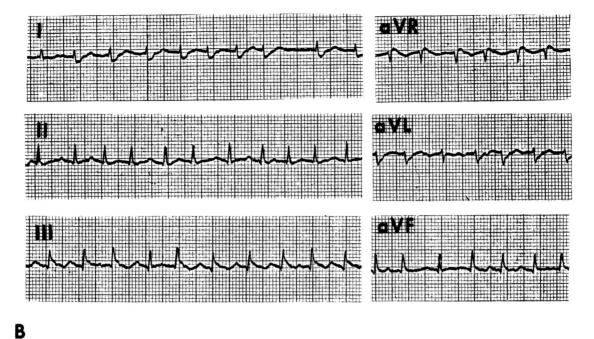

B

ECG I–47 (cont'd).   B. *Chaotic atrial tachycardia.* The P-waves may be quite subtle.

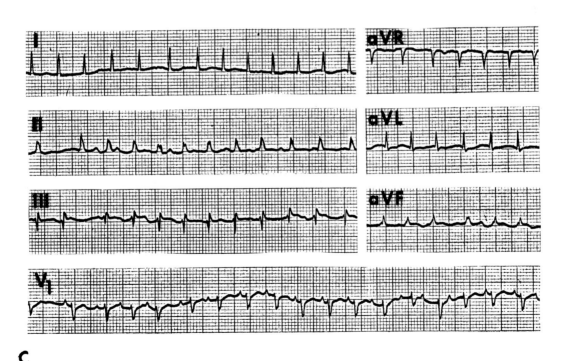

C

ECG I–47 (cont'd).   C. *Chaotic atrial tachycardia.*

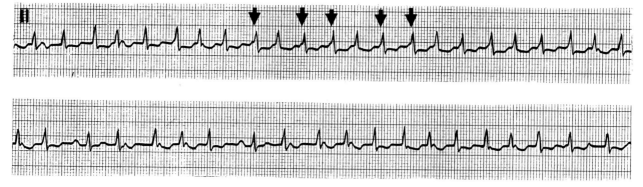

ECG I–48.   *Chaotic atrial tachycardia.* Many of the P-waves are buried within the QRS-complexes. Arrows point to a few of these P-waves.

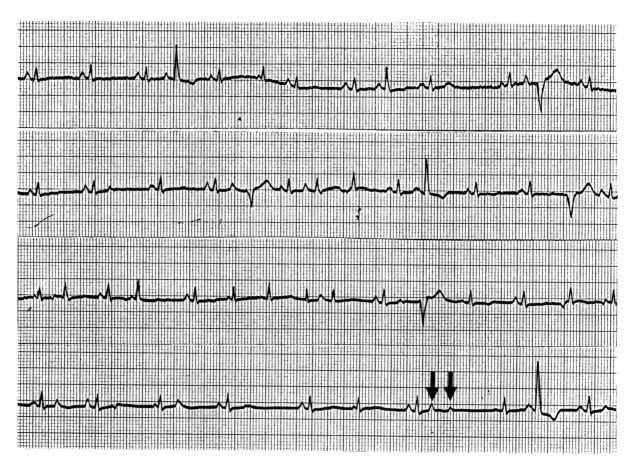

ECG I–49.   *Chaotic atrial tachycardia.* A number of the P-waves are conducted with functional aberration, or are nonconducted. The arrows point to a pair of nonconducted P-waves.

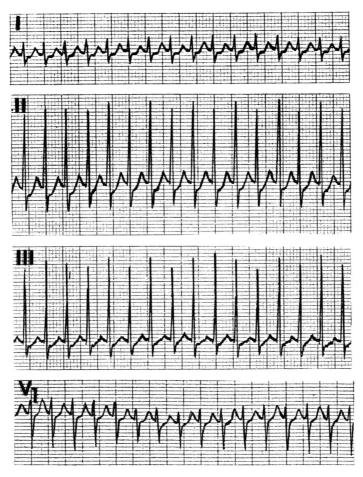

ECG I–50. *RSVT.* There is a regular supraventricular tachycardia at 240 bpm. No P-waves are visible. Mild QRS amplitude alternation, occasionally observed at heart rates of 220 bpm or greater, is present.

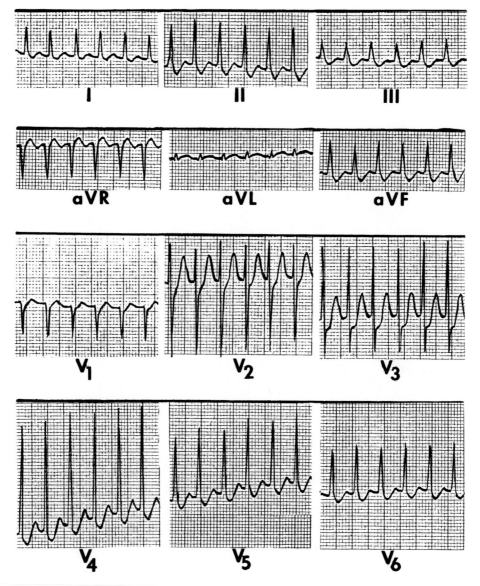

ECG I–51. *RSVT.* There is a regular supraventricular tachycardia at 188 bpm. The nadir of the T-waves in Leads I, II, III, and aVF are somewhat pointed, suggesting the superimposition of a retrograde-P-wave in each. In Lead V₁ the upright T-waves are also somewhat pointed—remember that retrograde-P-waves are usually upright in this lead.

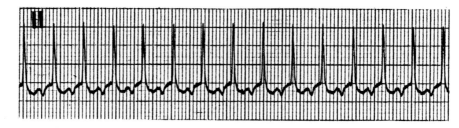

ECG I–52. *RSVT.* There is a regular supraventricular tachycardia at 188 bpm. Retrograde-P-waves occur in the middle of electrical diastole.

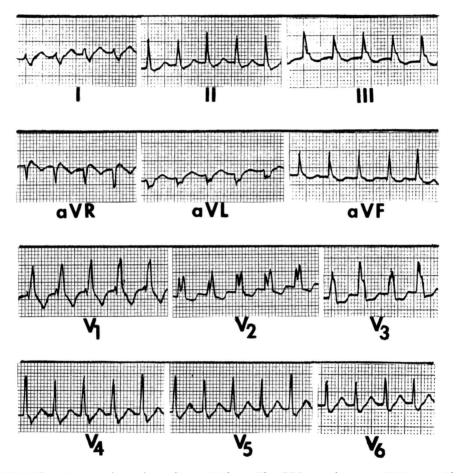

ECG I–53. *RSVT.* There is a regular tachycardia at 170 bpm. The QRS-complexes are 0.12 sec. wide, and have the morphology of classic RBBB. No P-waves are visible. (The small S-waves in Leads II, V₄ and V₅, and the small r-waves in aVR are part of the QRS-complex, and should not be mistaken for retrograde P-waves.)

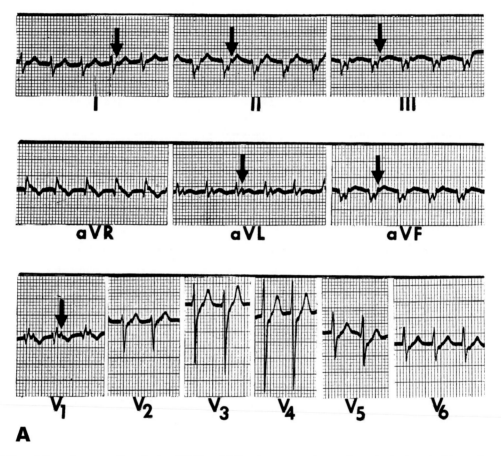

A

ECG I–54 (A and B are from a patient during RSVT and following conversion to sinus rhythm).   A. *RSVT*. There is a regular tachycardia at 160 bpm. The QRS-complexes have the morphology of RBBB and left anterior hemiblock. The small extra notch (arrow) at the end of each QRS-complex represents a retrograde-P-wave (negative in Leads II, III, and aVF, upright in V_1). It would be quite unusual for a QRS to demonstrate such complex morphology as an rSr's'r''s'' in Lead II, or an rsr's'r'' in Lead V_1. Up to the extra notch, the QRS-complexes are 0.12 sec. in duration.

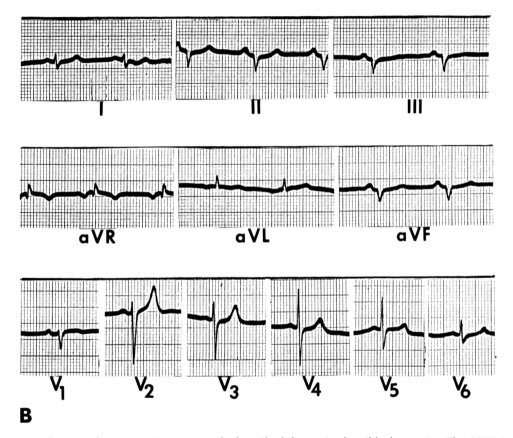

ECG I–54 (cont'd).   B. *After conversion to sinus rhythm.* The left anterior hemiblock remains. The RBBB is no longer present, suggesting it resulted from the faster rate (rate-related RBBB or sustained functional aberration). The retrograde-P-waves are also, of course, gone. (Stein, E. *The Electrocardiogram: A Self-Study Course in Clinical Electrocardiography.* Courtesy of W. B. Saunders Co., 1976.)

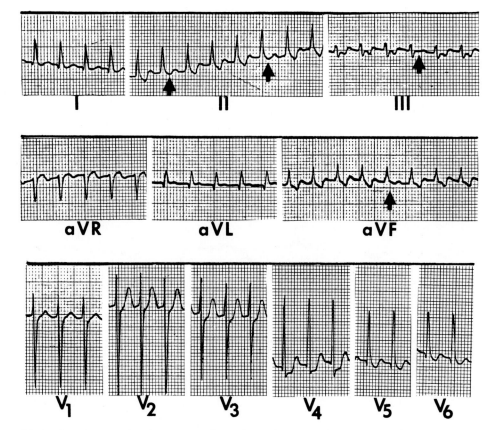

ECG I–55. *RSVT.* There is a regular supraventricular tachycardia at 188 bpm. Retrograde-P-waves intermittently fail to follow the QRS-complexes (arrows). This ECG illustrates that the atrium is not part of the reentry circuit, since the tachycardia continues despite failure to produce a retrograde-P-wave. It also follows that the reentry loop does not involve a Kent bundle as the retrograde pathway, since the impulse would have to traverse a portion of the atrium to reenter the A–V node after exiting from the Kent bundle. In summary, the reentry loop is located entirely within the A–V node.

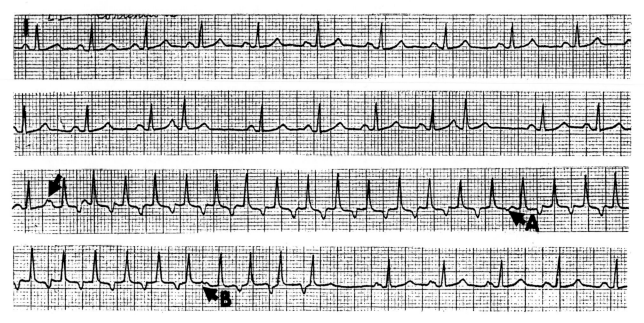

ECG I–56. *RSVT* triggered by a PAC. The basic rhythm is sinus. Three PACs are present. The third PAC (arrow) is conducted with sufficient A–V nodal delay (first-degree A–V block) to establish a reentry circuit. Note the retrograde-P-waves. What do A and B tell you about the site of reentry? Note the abrupt termination of the tachycardia. The electrocardiogram is from a continuous Lead I.

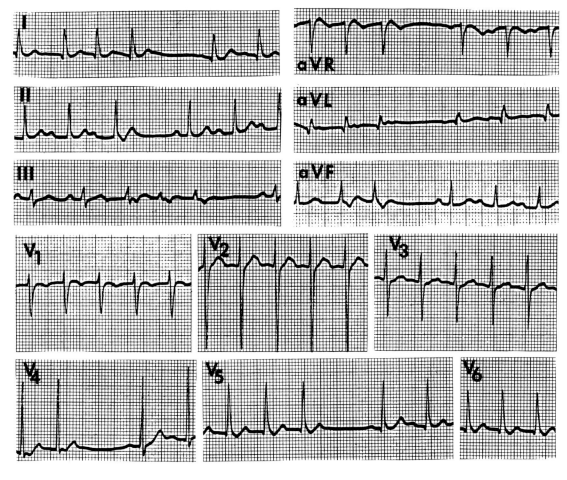

A

ECG I–57 (A and B are from the same patient). *RSVT triggered by A–V Wenckebach periods.* The basic rhythm is sinus tachycardia at 110 bpm. Progressive A–V nodal delay results in an atrial echo (arrows in rhythm strip, B), which may or may not herald sustained reentry. During the reentrant tachycardia (136 bpm), such retrograde P-waves follow each QRS. In Leads V_2 and V_3 (A), the upright retrograde-P-waves deform the T-waves. Following cessation of reentry, the sinus emerges after being reset by the preceding retrograde-P-wave.

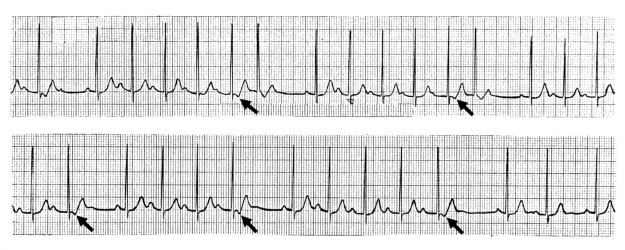

B

ECG I–57 (cont'd). B. Same patient as in A, from a continuous rhythm strip.

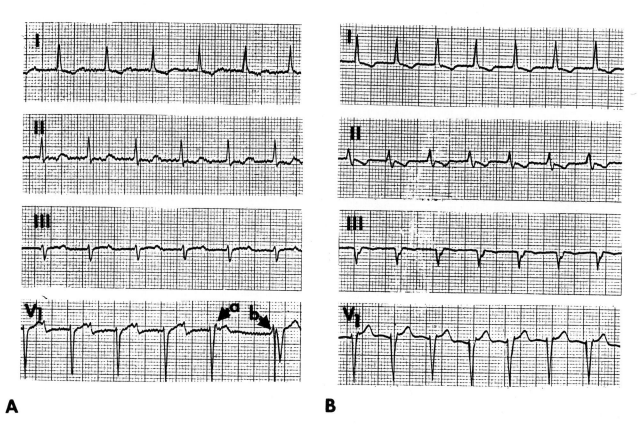

A   **B**

ECG I–58 (A, B and C are from the same patient).   *RSVT.* A. The rhythm is sinus with first-degree A–V block. Note the small upright deflection (a) following the fifth QRS-complex in Lead V_1. This represents either a nonconducted PAC or an atrial echo. (Even though the P–R interval does not measurably increase in V_1, remember that with such marked A–V delay already present, further prolongation of perhaps only several milliseconds may result in reentry.) The sinus is reset by this P-wave. Before this sinus-P-wave (b) can be fully inscribed, an artificial ventricular pacemaker escapes (note the pacemaker spike). B. Several months later the same patient is now found to be in a regular supraventricular tachycardia at 120 bpm. Although no P-waves are obvious, note the deeper "s-wave" in Leads II and III, as well as that same "r′" in V_1. That these deflections represent retrograde-P-waves is proven in the next electrocardiogram (C).

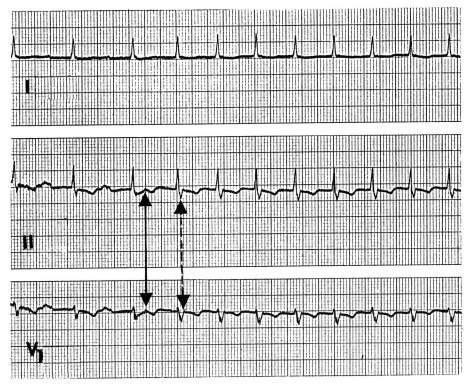

C

ECG I–58 (cont'd).   C. *RSVT.* That the deflections described in the preceding electrocardiogram (B) represent retrograde P-waves is proven here (simultaneous Leads I, II, and V_1). After two sinus beats with first-degree A–V block, a PAC (solid arrows) is conducted with additional A–V delay, resulting in an atrial echo (deeper "s" in II, new "r'" in V_1—broken arrows). Sustained reentry follows. The rate is relatively slow for an RSVT.

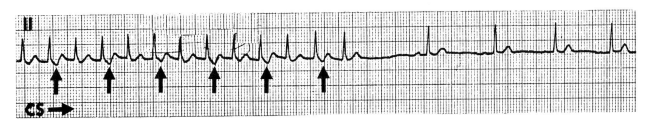

ECG I–59.   *RSVT with 2:1 retrograde atrial activation.* During vagal stimulation induced by carotid massage (CS), the A–V nodal reentrant loop continues for a time, but its connection to the atrium is blocked every other time. Note the slight increase in the last two R–R intervals before the tachycardia terminates. This slight slowing may represent slowing of conduction either around the reentrant loop or in the lower A–V nodal connection ("final common pathway") between the loop and the His bundle. The arrows indicate the retrograde-P-waves.

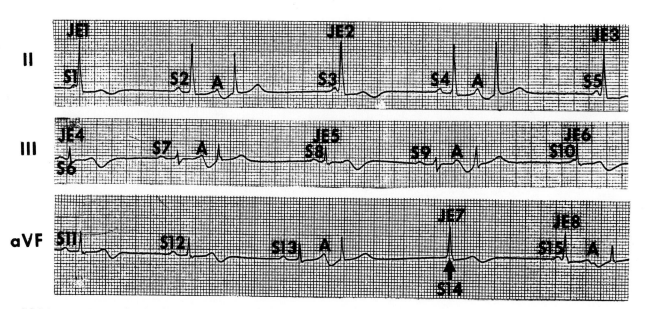

ECG I–60.   *Incomplete A–V dissociation.* In this tracing we note an irregular supraventricular rhythm. Antegrade-P-waves are present. Analysis of the atrial rhythm reveals sinus bradycardia (S) with frequent PACs (A). Note that within each lead the interval between a PAC and the subsequent sinus-P-wave is slightly longer than that between two sinus-P-waves. This small additional increment represents the time it takes for the PAC to enter the sinus node and reset it (review ECG I–16).

Two of the sinus-P-waves are partially buried in the QRS-complex (S1 and S10); one is completely buried (S14). These represent obvious instances of A–V dissociation. In each lead the sinus beats having longest constant P–R intervals represent conducted sinus beats (S2 and S4 in Lead II; S7 and S9 in Lead III; S11-S12-S13 in Lead aVF). Sinus-P-waves followed by shorter P–R intervals, even if they are not buried in the QRS, also represent instances of A–V dissociation (S3 and S5 in Lead II; S6 and S8 in Lead III; S15 in Lead aVF). All the PACs are conducted; their P–R intervals are longer than the P–R intervals of the conducted sinus beats, because, since they are so premature, the conducting system is still partially refractory.

The QRS-complexes at the times of A–V dissociation represent junctional escape beats (JE). Note that the longest R–R interval is that between two junctional escape beats (JE7-JE8). This represents the true junctional escape time (1510 msec., or a rate of 39/min.). Each of the other junctional escape beats follows a (conducted) PAC; the R–R intervals terminating in these other JEs are slightly shorter than the true JE time, since the junction is being reset at some point within the preceding P–R interval, at the instant the antegrade impulse from the PAC traverses the junctional area. By setting one's calipers for the true junctional rate (JE7–JE8), and measuring back one such cycle-length from JE2, 3, 5, 6, and 7, respectively, one can know exactly where in the preceding P–R interval this traversal and resetting of the junction occurred.

Finally, and most importantly, why are there periods of A–V dissociation? The junction (39/min.) is not accelerated. There is no A–V block (i.e., there are no P-waves in a position to capture which do not capture). The answer must be that the sinus is slow (40–46/min.). Whenever a PAC occurs, that small increment of time during which the sinus is entered and reset displaces the subsequent sinus-P to the right sufficiently for the junction to escape before that P-wave has a chance to conduct.

In conclusion, a proper description of this rhythm would be: sinus bradycardia with frequent PACs and periods of A–V dissociation with junctional escape beats (incomplete A–V dissociation). The junction is not accelerated, and there is no evidence of A–V block.

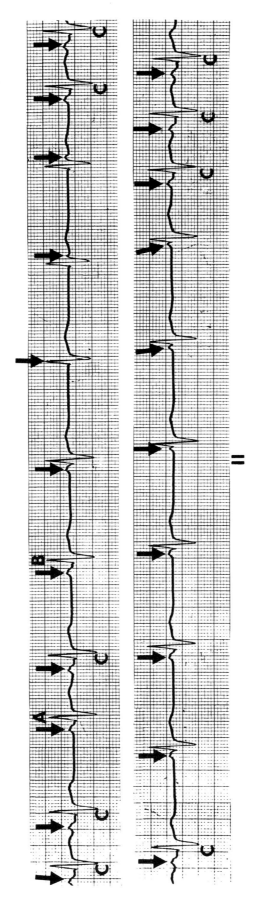

ECG I–61. *Incomplete A–V dissociation.* Marked sinus arrhythmia is present (arrows). During periods of sinus slowing, a junctional escape rhythm emerges at a rate of 47–50 bpm, producing A–V dissociation. A–V block is not present, since all P-waves in a position to capture do so (C). The identity of beats A and B is problematical. While they may be junctional escape beats, they could well be sinus captures, since there is a tendency toward slightly shorter P–R intervals at slower rates (examine the P–R intervals of the last 3 sinus captures).

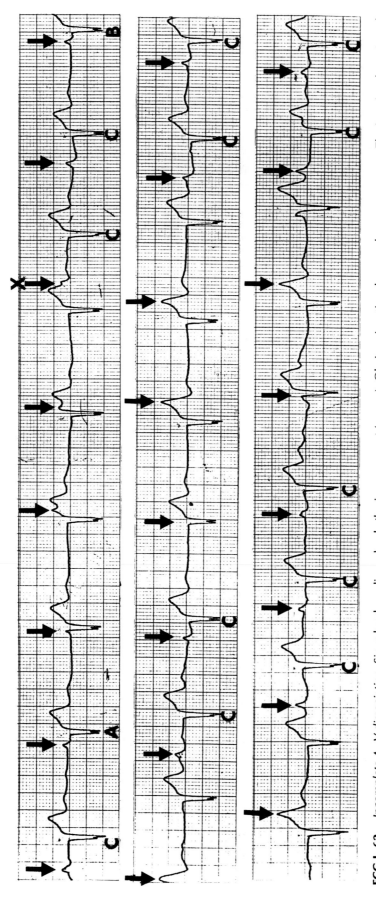

ECG I–62. *Incomplete A–V dissociation.* Sinus bradycardia and arrhythmia are present. Obvious junctional escape beats are present (arrows). The junctional rate is 49 bpm in the top strip, but "warms up" to 59 bpm by the bottom strip. The QRS-complexes representing sinus captures are marked C; each is preceded by a P–R interval between 0.22 and 0.60 sec. The P–R intervals of the capture vary inversely with the closeness of the P-wave to the previous beat (i.e., with the "R–P interval" of the previous beat). A–V block is not present, since all P-waves in a position to capture do so. In fact, beats such as X, within the T-wave of the previous beat, yet able to capture, indicate excellent A–V conduction. As in ECG I–61, beats A and B may be either junctional escape beats or sinus captures.

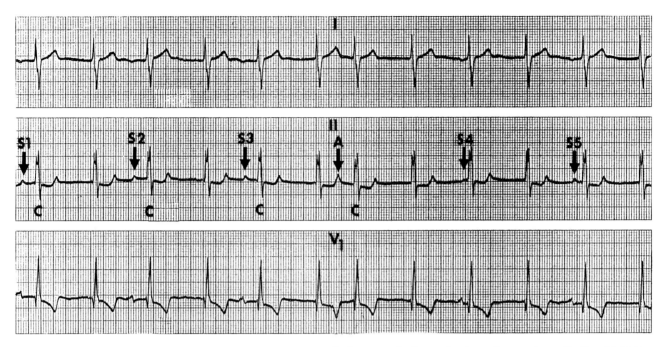

ECG I–63. *Incomplete A–V dissociation.* The underlying rhythm is marked sinus bradycardia at 33 bpm (S). One PAC (A) is present, and appropriately resets the sinus. Obvious junctional escape beats are present; the junctional escape rate is 65/min. There are four antegrade captures (C), three from the sinus (S1, S2 and S3) and one from the PAC. A–V block is not present; S4 and S5 would have captured if they hadn't been preempted by the junction. In this ECG, the causes of the A–V dissociation are (1) slowing of the sinus, and (2) slight acceleration of the junction. These simultaneous Leads I, II, and V₁ are on double standard.

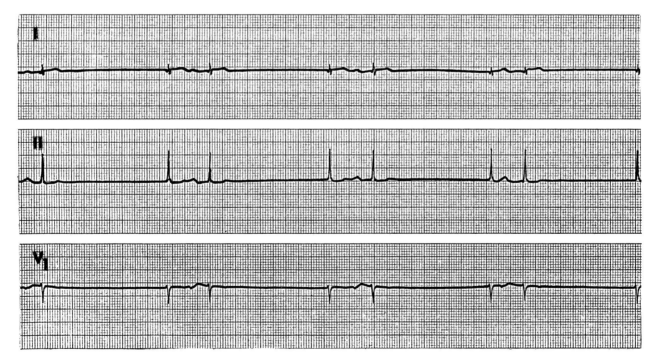

ECG I–64. *Incomplete A–V dissociation.* Marked sinus bradycardia at 23–25 bpm is present. Following each sinus capture, a slow junctional escape beat emerges; the escape rate is approximately 32 bpm. A bigeminal pattern is thus produced, with the sinus captures comprising the "premature beats." Simultaneous Leads I, II and V₁ have been recorded.

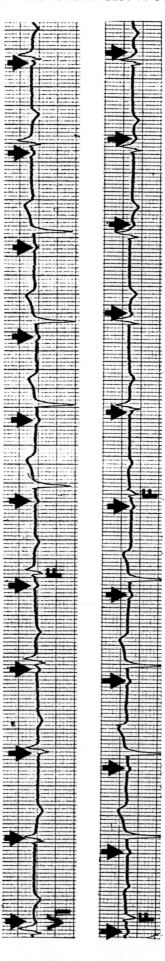

ECG I-65. *Incomplete A–V dissociation.* The sinus rate varies from 60–68 bpm (arrows). During periods of sinus slowing, an accelerated subjunctional rhythm emerges at a rate of 61–67 bpm, producing A–V dissociation. The escape pacemaker is located in the proximal left bundle branch; the QRSs therefore have a RBBB pattern. Since the escape pacemaker is located below the bifurcation of the bundle of His, fusions between it and sinus captures can occur. Three such beats (F) are, in fact, present.

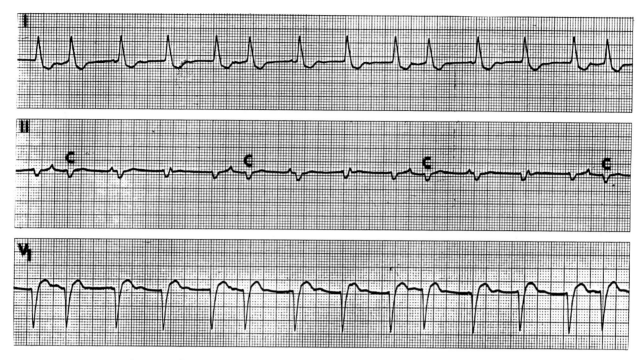

ECG I–66. *Incomplete A–V dissociation.* The underlying sinus rate is 66 bpm. A–V dissociation is caused by an accelerated junctional rhythm at 84 bpm. No A–V block is present; the four P-waves in a position to produce captures do so (C). LBBB is present in the sinus captures as well as the junctional beats, indicating the latter do not arise below the bifurcation of the His bundle (review ECG I–65). Simultaneous Leads I, II, and V₁ have been recorded.

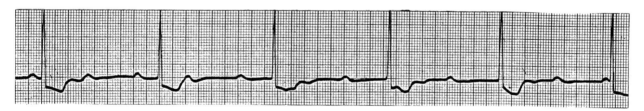

ECG I–67. *Complete A–V dissociation.* The sinus rate is 75 bpm. There is a slow junctional escape rhythm at 33/min. No captures occur, even though many of the P-waves ought to have done so. The sinus is not slow, nor is the junction accelerated. The cause of the A–V dissociation is therefore advanced A–V block. (Stein, E. *The Electrocardiogram: A Self-Study Course in Clinical Electrocardiography.* Courtesy of W. B. Saunders Co., 1976.)

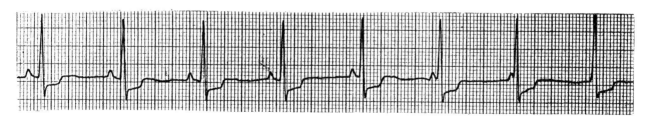

ECG I–68. *Complete A–V dissociation.* The sinus rate is 65 bpm. There is an accelerated junctional rhythm at 67 bpm. Since the junction is faster than the sinus, A–V dissociation occurs. Although no captures are present in the rhythm strip, *the presence of A–V block cannot be ascertained,* since no P-wave which is not preempted by the junction is seen. (Stein, E. *The Electrocardiogram: A Self-Study Course in Clinical Electrocardiography.* Courtesy of W. B. Saunders Co., 1976.)

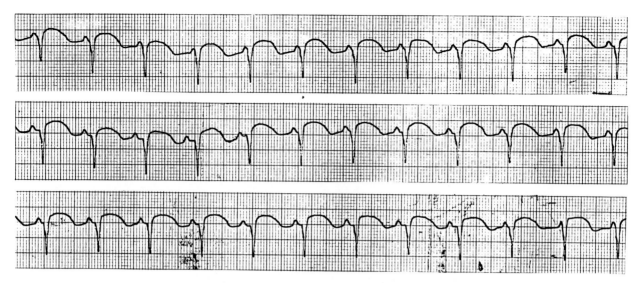

ECG I–69. *Isorhythmic A–V dissociation.* Both the sinus and junction fire at 87 bpm. Although the P–R intervals vary, the sinus-P-waves never fully merge into the QRS-complexes. Note how perusal of the first four beats of the middle strip might lead to the erroneous impression of sinus rhythm. No captures (early QRSs) are, in fact, present. The cause of the complete A–V dissociation is acceleration of the junction. As in ECG I–68, the presence of A–V block cannot be ascertained.

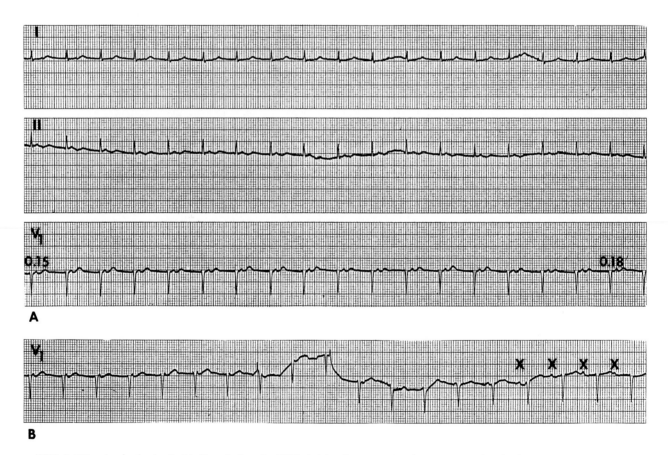

ECG I–70. *Isorhythmic A–V dissociation.* In ECG A (simultaneous Leads I, II, V₁), the rhythm appears to be sinus tachycardia (at 100 bpm) with first-degree A–V block; the P-waves are upright in Leads II and V₁, flat in I. Careful perusal, however, reveals that the "R–P interval" of the last beat is slightly larger than that of the first. Additional rhythm strip (V₁ shown below—B) reveals complete A–V dissociation to indeed be present. The causes of the A–V dissociation are (1) acceleration of the junction, and (2) A–V block (since none of the P-waves labeled X produces captures).

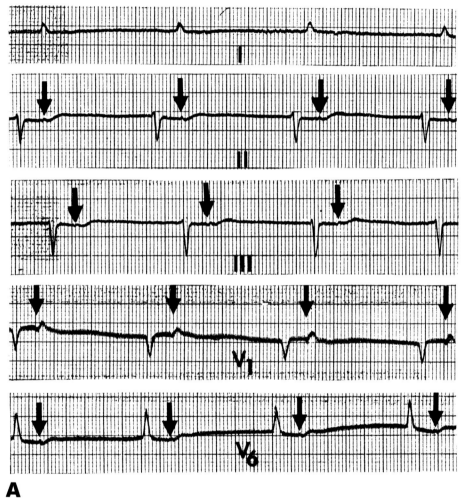

A

ECG I–71. *Junctional rhythm with 1:1 V–A conduction.* A. Slow junctional rhythm (40–44 bpm). Retrograde-P-waves (arrows) follow each QRS. Since each retrograde-P-wave resets the sinus, the underlying sinus rate must be less than 40 bpm.

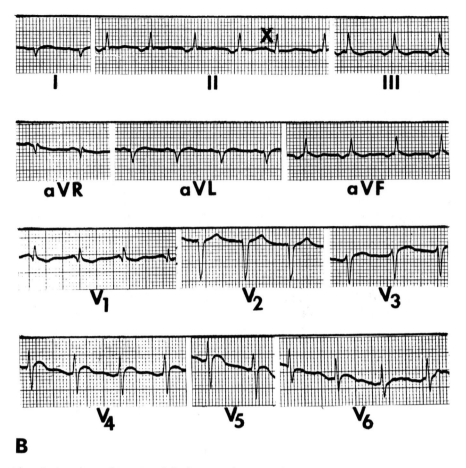

B

ECG I–71 (cont'd).   B. Accelerated junctional rhythm (110 bpm). Each QRS is preceded by a retrograde-P-wave; the P–R interval is 0.12 sec. A single PAC (X) is present.

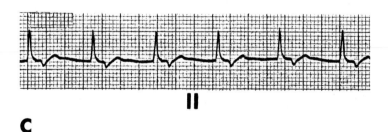

C

ECG I–71 (cont'd).   C. Accelerated junctional rhythm (88 bpm). A retrograde-P-wave follows each QRS.

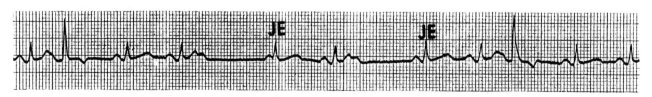

ECG I–72.   *Junctional escape beats (JE) unmasked by nonconducted PACs.* The basic rhythm is sinus. There are two PACs conducted with functional aberration and two nonconducted PACs. The pauses following the latter, during which the sinus is reset, are terminated by junctional escape beats having normal escape times of 1.16 and 1.09 sec. (corresponding to 52 and 55 bpm, respectively).

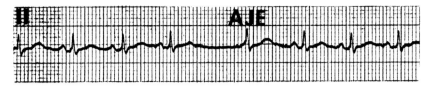

ECG I–73. *Accelerated junctional escape beat (AJE) unmasked by a nonconducted PAC.* The AJE falls on the apex of the reset sinus-P-wave. The junctional escape time of 0.80 sec., corresponding to 75 bpm, is accelerated. The accelerated junctional escape time is the only manifestation of digitalis toxicity in this ECG. Note that if the PAC had not occurred, the accelerated junctional pacemaker would not have become manifest until it exceeded the sinus rate of 115 bpm, representing a far greater degree of digitalis poisoning.

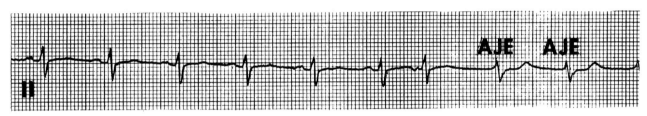

A

ECG I–74. *Accelerated junctional rhythm (AJR) unmasked by extrasystoles.* A. AJR at 80 bpm unmasked by a PAC. Note the sinus rate of 83 bpm.

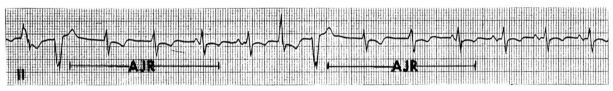

B

ECG I–74 (cont'd). B. AJR at 77 bpm unmasked by PVCs. Following the paired PVCs, a three-beat run of AJR emerges. Note the sinus rate of 87 bpm.

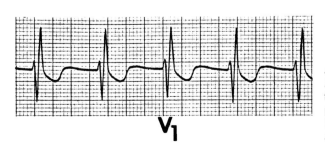

ECG I–75. *Accelerated junctional rhythm with RBBB vs. accelerated subjunctional rhythm arising from the left bundle branch.* The rate is 86 bpm. There is either 1:1 V–A conduction, with the retrograde-P-waves buried within the QRS-complexes, or underlying atrial fibrillation. A previous ECG may help differentiate both the location of the escaping pacemaker as well as the underlying atrial rhythm. Can you tell how?

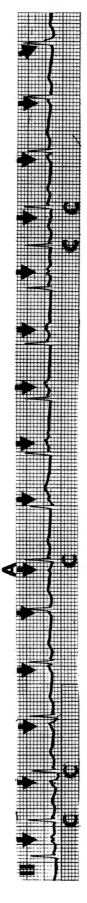

ECG I–76. *Incomplete A–V dissociation.* The basic rhythm is wandering atrial pacemaker (arrows). Note the varying P-wave morphology. One PAC (A) is present. (Note A comes early and resets the next atrial depolarization.) There are periods of accelerated junctional rhythm with A–V dissociation. The basic atrial rate is approximately 94 bpm; the junctional rate is 100 bpm. As in previous examples, the (accelerated) junctional escape beats terminate the longest R–R intervals present. Shorter R–R intervals are terminated by antegrade captures (C). All P-waves in a position to capture do so, excluding A–V block. The cause of the A–V dissociation is acceleration of the junction.

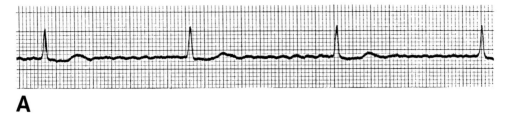

A

ECG I–77. *Progression of digitalis toxicity in atrial fibrillation (AF).* A. The baseline is AF. The R–R intervals are regular, indicating complete A–V nodal block with a slow junctional escape rhythm at 38 bpm.

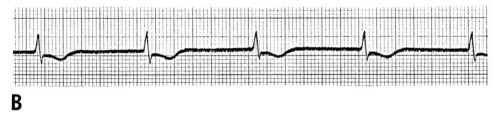

B

ECG I–77 (cont'd).   B. With a further increase in the serum digitalis level, the junctional rate picks up to 50 bpm. (A and B. Stein, E. *The Electrocardiogram: A Self-Study Course in Clinical Electrocardiography.* Courtesy of W. B. Saunders Co., 1976.)

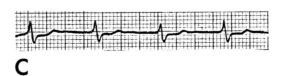

C

ECG I–77 (cont'd).   C. With a further increase in the serum digitalis level, the junction has now accelerated to 85 bpm.

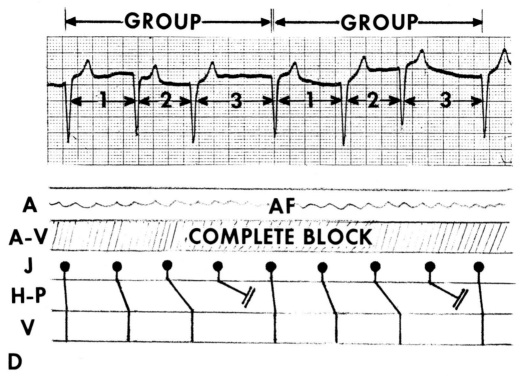

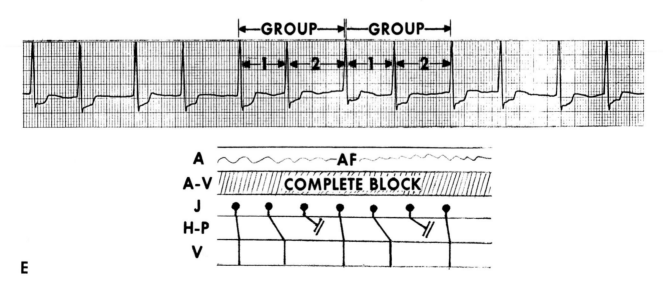

ECG I–77 (cont'd).   D. The rhythm has now become *regularly irregular. Group beating* is present, indicating the presence of Wenckebach conduction. Note the replication of each R–R interval of the group. The junctional rate has now reached 86 bpm. There is such advanced digitalis poisoning that a *second level of block* (of 4:3 Wenckebach type) has developed between the accelerated junctional escape pacemaker and the ventricles (H–V block). This poisoning of the His-Purkinje system is frequently a pre-terminal event. The junctional rate may be calculated by dividing one group of three beats and a pause by four, since one knows that there is a fourth junctional pacemaker depolarization which has failed to reach the ventricles to make a QRS. The underlying rhythm is still AF, with complete A–V block above the junction, in the A–V node. A fatal mistake would be to confuse the *regular irregularity* of the group beating with the *irregular irregularity* of simple AF. (Reproduced with permission from Kastor, J., and Yurchak, P.: Recognition of digitalis intoxication in the presence of atrial fibrillation. Ann. Intern. Med., *67*:1045, 1967.)

A = Atria; A–V = A–V Node; J = Junction; H–P = His-Purkinje; V = Ventricles; AF = Atrial Fibrillation

ECG I–77 (cont'd).   E. Group beating consisting of a repetitive bigeminal rhythm is now present. The junctional rate is now 119 bpm. H–V conduction has decreased to 3:2. Such a patient is so digitalis-toxic that ventricular fibrillation could supervene at any time.

A = Atria; A–V = A–V Node; J = Junction; H–P = His-Purkinje; V = Ventricles; AF = Atrial Fibrillation

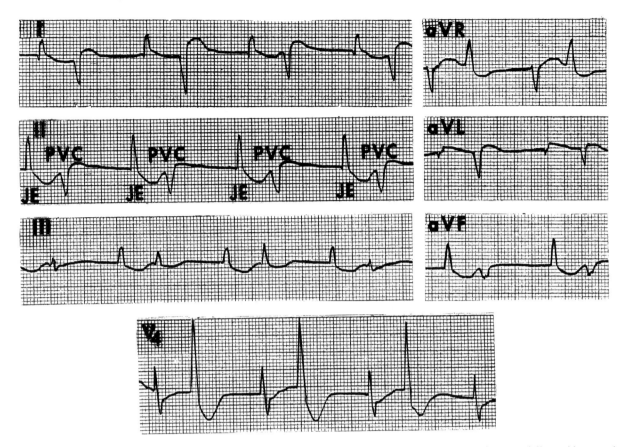

ECG I–78. In this tracing we note a repetitive bigeminal rhythm consisting of a supraventricular QRS followed by a wide bizarre QRS (PVC). No P-waves are present. Ignoring the PVCs for the moment, the rhythm is atrial fibrillation with regular QRSs; therefore, there is complete heart block at the A–V nodal level, and a junctional escape rhythm. Because there are always PVCs in bigeminy (i.e., never one junctional beat following another), we cannot determine the true junctional rate. It may be the *apparent* junctional rate, *twice* the apparent junctional rate, or a rate *intermediate* between the two.

True junctional rate = apparent junctional rate: PVC does not significantly retrogradely penetrate the conducting system.

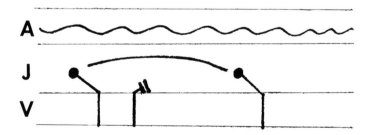

True junctional rate = 2 × apparent junctional rate: PVC has significant concealed retrograde penetration of the conducting system, but does not reach the junction. The subsequent junctional impulse finds the conducting system refractory and is, therefore, blocked.

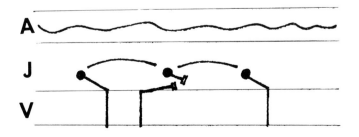

Apparent junctional rate < true junctional rate < 2 × apparent junctional rate: PVC has concealed retrograde conduction back to the junction, which is reset.

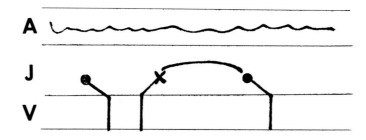

In summary, this rhythm can be described as follows: atrial fibrillation with complete A–V (nodal) block, junctional escape rhythm at 49/min. which may actually be accelerated junctional rhythm up to 98/min., and PVCs in bigeminy. This rhythm is digitalis-toxic. The true junctional rate is important only in that in digitalis-toxic junctional acceleration, the degree of acceleration is usually proportional to the degree of intoxication (review ECG series I–77, A–E). The unifocal, multiforme PVC morphology is also frequently seen in digitalis toxicity. Note the marked digitalis ST-T effect, indicating that the patient is indeed taking digitalis.

A = Atria; J = Junction; V = Ventricles.

Heart Block* and Other Bradyarrhythmias

INTRODUCTION

The normal A–V conducting system consists of the *A–V node* and the *His-Purkinje system.* The latter begins with the *bundle of His,* a short structure which divides into right and left bundle branches. The *right bundle branch* runs down the right side of the interventricular septum. The *left bundle branch* almost immediately divides into an *anterior fascicle,* running down the left side of the septum, and a *posterior fascicle,* a much broader structure which fans out posteriorly and inferiorly. The right bundle branch along with the two divisions of the left form the *trifascicular system.* Innervation of the interventricular septum is *via* one or more septal fascicles arising from the main left bundle branch, or from its anterior or posterior divisions. The trifascicular system arborizes into an extensive *Purkinje network,* which innervates the ventricular myocardium.

In this section, block of the A–V conducting system, both in the A–V node and in the infranodal system will be discussed. In addition, other bradyarrhythmias, namely, those involving the S–A node, will also be covered. Before embarking on a discussion of A–V block, let us discuss the Wenckebach phenomenon.

Wenckebach Conduction

Wenckebach conduction is characterized by progressive delay of conduction culminating in the failure of a single beat to conduct (single dropped

beat). Wenckebach periods therefore have conduction ratios of $(n + 1) : n$. While Wenckebach conduction occurs commonly in the A–V node (i.e., A–V Wenckebach periods), the phenomenon may occur in any conducting tissue of the heart (see Table II–1). In *typical* Wenckebach periods, the conduction times show progressive increase, but the intervals between the beats which are produced show progressive *decrease* prior to the drop. This occurs because the *increment* of delay of each beat over that of the previous beat progressively *decreases* (see Figure II–1). The behavior of appropriate intervals in various typical Wenckebach periods is illustrated in Table II–2. In typical Wenckebach periods, the pause containing the dropped beat is less than the sum of the two preceding inter-beat intervals. In addition, the interval after the pause is longer than that preceding the pause (except, of course, in 3:2 Wenckebach periods, in which they are identical). These characteristics are also illustrated in Figure II–1. In typical Wenckebach periods, those periods having the

TABLE II–1. Wenckebach Conduction.

Common
1. In the A–V node (A–V Wenckebach)
2. Surrounding the S–A node (S–A Wenckebach)
3. In the His-Purkinje system (H–V Wenckebach) associated with accelerated junctional rhythm (advanced digitalis toxicity, or, rarely, acute myocardial infarction)

Uncommon
1. Surrounding an ectopic atrial pacemaker (S′–A Wenckebach)
2. In the bundle branches
3. Surrounding a parasystolic focus

---

*In this book, heart block, a commonly used term in clinical practice, refers to atrioventricular (A–V) block.

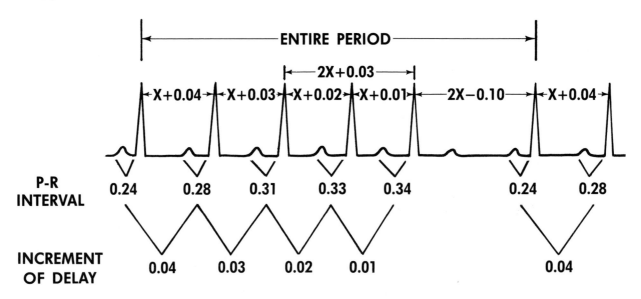

X = P–P INTERVAL (CONSTANT)

Figure II–1. Typical A–V Wenckebach period.

same conducting ratios (e.g., 5:4, 4:3, etc.) precisely replicate each other; that is, the length of each of the respective intervals, as well as that of the entire Wenckebach period,* are identical. In typical A–V Wenckebach periods, one can directly measure the underlying sinus rate, since it is equal to the (constant) P-wave rate. In S–A and H–V Wenckebach periods, however, the true sinus and junctional rates, respectively, must be calculated. One takes the length of the entire Wenckebach period and divides by the number of P-waves plus one or R-waves plus one, respectively, contained within that cycle. The true sinus or junctional rate, respectively, should be identical when calculated from typical S–A or H–V Wenckebach periods of different conduction ratios. The identical underlying pacemaker rates for different ratio cycles, as well as the precise replication of similar ratio cy-

cles, can be used to differentiate true S–A and H–V Wenckebach periods from sinus arrhythmia and junctional arrhythmia (or atrial fibrillation with an irregular response), respectively, in cases where at times the latter may mimic the "group beating" of the former. True "group beating," that is, repetitive clusters of beats with progressively decreasing intervals followed by a pause, often can be spotted at a glance, and usually indicates the presence of some type of Wenckebach period. One then examines the rhythm in more detail to ascertain its nature.

A–V NODAL BLOCK

Block of conduction in the A–V node may be first-degree (1°), second-degree (2°), or advanced. First-degree A–V block is characterized by P–R interval prolongation, reflecting A–V nodal delay. Such P–R intervals range from 0.21 to 0.60 sec. Second-degree A–V nodal block, or Mobitz Type I

---

*The entire Wenckebach period is measured from the first beat of the sequence to the beat terminating the long pause.

TABLE II–2. Characteristics of Various Typical Wenckebach Periods.

Name	Constant	Progressively Increases	Progressively Decreases Before Drop
S–A Wenckebach	S–A nodal discharge*	Sinus-atrium interval*	P–P**
A–V Wenckebach	P–P	P–R	R–R
H–V Wenckebach	Junctional pacemaker discharge*	Junction-ventricle interval*	R–R

*Not visible on the ECG.
**R–R interval decrease secondarily follows P–P decrease, unless A–V block is present.

A–V block, is characterized by A–V Wenckebach periods. These may be *typical* or *atypical*. In typical A–V Wenckebach periods, there is a progressive increase in the P–R intervals and a progressive decrease in the R–R intervals before the pause containing the dropped beat. In such cycles the greatest increment of delay of A–V conduction occurs at the beginning of the sequence. In atypical A–V Wenckebach periods, the greatest change may occur in the middle or at the end of the sequence.* Factors promoting atypicality are: (1) long sequences, (2) vagal surges, (3) underlying sinus arrhythmia and changing vagal tone. In the latter two circumstances, the increasing P–R intervals are accompanied by lengthening P–P intervals, since both reflect heightened vagal tone.** In significant sinus arrhythmia, although the P–R intervals may lengthen and shorten throughout the sequence, the Wenckebach phenomenon may still be inferred since the trend is toward longer P–R intervals at the end of the sequence than at the beginning (see ECG II–8). Occasionally a sudden vagal surge may be mistaken on superficial inspection for a *sudden dropped beat* (Mobitz Type II block). Careful inspection reveals a slight lengthening of the P–R interval before the dropped beat, a longer P–R interval before the dropped beat than after, and a slight increase in the P–P interval at the time of the drop. Whatever the reasons for being atypical, the R–R intervals do not progressively shorten to form the group-beating cluster, as is found in typical A–V Wenckebach periods.

Changing P–R intervals may also occur as a manifestation of *dual pathway conduction* (see ECG IV–16). Under these circumstances, there are two distinct P–R intervals, with either random or alternating changeovers between the two; during periods of alternation, one set of beats may occasionally manifest an A–V Wenckebach period, while the alternate set of P–R intervals remains *constant*. In contradistinction, occasionally, beats demonstrating progressive Wenckebach conduction alternate with *nonconducted* beats. Such *alternating Wenckebach periods* indicate bilevel A–V block, and will be discussed later.

A–V Wenckebach periods may be altered by still other arrhythmias. Premature ventricular beats (PVCs) may occur at any point in the cycle. A premature atrial beat (PAC) may occur close to the dropped beat; *two* nonconducted P-waves may re-

sult. An A–V Wenckebach sequence may be terminated by an *atrial echo;* such a retrograde-P-wave preempts the next anticipated sinus-P-wave. Of course, one or more reentry beats (i.e., ventricular echoes) may follow. Finally, *S–A Wenckebach periods* may coexist with A–V Wenckebach periods. If the conducting ratio of the latter exceeds that of the former (i.e., 5:4 A–V *vs.* 4:3 S–A), the P-wave itself drops before the A–V Wenckebach sequence is completed; under these circumstances, no nonconducted P-wave occurs.

The beat terminating an A–V or S–A Wenckebach pause is usually another sinus beat. However, depending on the length of the pause as well as the escape time of the subsidiary pacemaker, a *junctional escape beat* may emerge.

BLOCK OF RETROGRADE A–V NODAL CONDUCTION

During junctional, idioventricular, or artificial ventricular pacemaker rhythm, retrograde conduction to the atria may occur. Such conduction may be 1:1, 2:1, or, if intermediate, of Wenckebach type. Such *V–A Wenckebach periods* are characterized by progressive increase in the R-to-retrograde-P intervals (the "R–P intervals"), culminating in a dropped retrograde-P-wave. Of course, just as with antegrade A–V nodal conduction, reentry may occur, so that the sequence is terminated by a ventricular echo (which also may be followed by additional reentry beats).

INFRA-NODAL BLOCK

Block of conduction below the A–V node occurs as a result of His bundle block or bilateral bundle branch block (bilateral BBB). Simple delay of infra-nodal conduction occurs, but is usually in the order of 10 to 50 msec. (i.e., usually less than one small box on the ECG); although the presence of infra-nodal delay cannot be ascertained on the surface ECG, if the P–R interval is significantly prolonged (> 0.24 sec.), all or most of the delay is A–V nodal. 2° block below the A–V node, or Mobitz Type II A–V block, is characterized by one or more *sudden dropped beats*. There is no measurable antecedent increase in the P–R interval.* Of course, all the P–R intervals may be prolonged because of coexisting A–V nodal delay; however, no further increase occurs before the dropped beat. In A–V nodal block, a slowing of the sinus rate often coincides with the dropped beat. This is

---

*Such atypical periods therefore do not manifest "group beating."
**In significant sinus arrhythmia or changing vagal tone, the P–R intervals may vary without the production of a dropped beat.

---

*Electrophysiologic studies have revealed that the H–V interval (i.e., infra-nodal conduction time) may increase by 5–10 msec. immediately before the dropped beat, but this is too small to be measurable on the surface ECG.

because heightened vagal activity is responsible for both. In infra-nodal block, the dropped beat or beats is frequently associated with an *increase* in the sinus rate, and, in fact, is often induced by exercise. This is because the faster sinus rate presents more impulses to the diseased conducting system; the reduced vagal tone is of no benefit, since the vagal fibers do not reach beyond the upper A–V junction. Of course, atrial pacing may induce either A–V nodal and/or infra-nodal block, since vagal tone is unaltered by the artificial pacing. Mobitz II block may also be provoked by a spontaneously occurring PAC or PVC.

Bilateral BBB is the most common location of infra-nodal block, although there is evidence that the His bundle, whose fibers may be predestined to join the right or left bundle branches, may be involved as well. It is not uncommon to have one or multiple changing BBB patterns in the conducted beats of an individual manifesting infra-nodal block. If the QRS-complexes are narrow, however, the site of infra-nodal block is presumed to be in the His bundle.

OTHER ASPECTS OF INFRA-NODAL BLOCK

Although 2° A–V block in the His-Purkinje system is characterized by Mobitz Type II block, the Wenckebach phenomenon may also occur. The usual circumstances involve acute myocardial infarction (MI) or digitalis toxicity, resulting in complete A–V nodal block and accelerated junctional rhythm. As the junction becomes more accelerated, junctional-ventricular (H–V) block of Wenckebach type may develop. As in the case of all typical Wenckebach periods, "group beating" is present.* Although clinically uncommon, Wenckebach conduction in a bundle branch may occur. In such cases, the QRS-complexes progress from normal to incomplete right or incomplete left BBB to complete BBB morphology. If, at the time of the complete BBB, the contralateral bundle is also completely blocked, a dropped beat occurs (see ECG II–25).

A complete BBB pattern, producing a QRS-complex of 0.12 sec. or more duration, may reflect either true 3° (i.e., complete) block or severe slowing (1° block) of that bundle. In either case, completely asynchronous activation of the ventricles occurs, hence, the 0.12 sec. QRS. When 3° block of a bundle is added to pre-existing 3° block of the other

bundle, A–V conduction is interrupted. When severe 1° block of the right bundle is complicated by either relatively more severe slowing or 3° block of the left bundle, the ECG will change from complete RBBB to complete LBBB *with slight P–R prolongation* (by approximately 0.03 to 0.06 sec.). The P–R prolongation occurs because A–V conduction must now proceed exclusively through a bundle(s) which has severe slowing. If severe 1° block of a bundle is complicated by equally severe slowing in the other bundle, the result is a *normal QRS-complex* with slight P–R prolongation. The QRS normalizes, because, with equal slowing, the activation of the ventricles is now synchronous. The beats of patients who develop Mobitz II block on the basis of bilateral BBB always manifest a complete BBB pattern. It is not uncommon for such patients to have varying BBB morphologies at different times or occurring together. Complete RBBB and complete LBBB, complete RBBB with left anterior and posterior hemiblock, or any combination of the foregoing may occur. A shift from one BBB pattern to another or to a normal QRS with P–R prolongation, or the addition of Wenckebach conduction in one bundle to pre-existing block of the other, all bespeak severe bilateral bundle disease, and carry a high risk of 2° or advanced heart block.

Finally, it must be pointed out that Mobitz II block could be mimicked by a concealed discharge of a junctional pacemaker. An early junctional premature beat (PJC) coming after a long R–R interval may encounter functional trifascicular block in its antegrade conduction and complete A–V nodal block in its retrograde conduction. Since it cannot produce either a QRS or retrograde-P-wave, it is invisible on the surface ECG. If the next sinus-P-wave follows in close order, it encounters a zone of refractoriness at the site of the junctional depolarization and cannot conduct. What appears to be a *sudden dropped beat* is seen. Such a "pseudo-Mobitz II" phenomenon is diagnosed when a single dropped beat occurs in an asymptomatic patient who has a relatively slow heart rate and frequent PJCs. Of course, if an intracardiac His bundle electrogram is obtained, the concealed junctional discharge will appear as an extra His spike antecedent to the dropped beat.

ADVANCED HEART BLOCK

A–V block in which the conducting ratio is 2:1 or greater is considered advanced heart block. Although the term "3°" or "complete heart block" is frequently applied to advanced A–V block in which no captures occur, it is in a strict sense a misnomer in most cases, since one can never prove

---

*If the underlying atrial rhythm is sinus, nonparoxysmal atrial tachycardia (NPAT), or atrial flutter—rather than AF—the homologous beats of each Wenckebach sequence have no constant relationship to their antecedent P-waves (review Section I, pp. 19-20 and see ECG II–46A).

that, had the junctional or ventricular escape beat not occurred, the next sinus-P-wave would not have captured. At any rate, advanced heart block may result from a progression of *either A–V nodal or infranodal* 2° A–V block (i.e., from Mobitz I or Mobitz II block, respectively). When faced with an ECG showing advanced heart block, one must diligently search the rhythm strip for *two consecutively conducted P-waves* in order to ascertain whether the block is A–V nodal or infranodal. If there is an increase in the P–R interval before the dropped beat, the site of block is in the A–V node. Also, if one searches portions of the rhythm strip remote to the period of advanced heart block, or if one has another rhythm strip taken shortly before, and A–V Wenckebach periods are found, one can infer the A–V node as the site of block.

Fixed 2:1, 3:1, etc., block may be A–V nodal or infranodal, regardless of the presence of a BBB pattern or unvarying P–R prolongation of the conducted beats.* Again, one requires two consecutively conducted beats, or A–V Wenckebach periods elsewhere, to make the diagnosis. Unless one is certain of the clinical circumstances, one should not administer atropine to the patient with fixed-ratio advanced heart block. If one is dealing with known digitalis intoxication, acute inferior/dorsal wall MI, or congenital complete heart block, one already knows that the site of block is the A–V node. Atropine will either improve A–V conduction (except in the case of congenital block) and/or will increase the rate of the junctional pacemaker. In the case of acute anterior wall MI, or if the clinical circumstances are unknown, the likelihood of infra-nodal block is high; atropine may *worsen* the block by increasing the atrial rate.

In advanced heart block, when the conducting ratio is 2:1 (or in "complete" heart block when the atrial rate is approximately twice that of the escaping pacemaker), "ventriculophasic effect" may occur. On the ECG, one observes that the P–P intervals *surrounding* each QRS are *shorter* than those between the QRSs. The mechanism is as follows: Because of the heart block, the heart rate is slow. Each ventricular systole therefore occurs with a maximally filled left ventricle. The increased stroke volume of such beats is sensed by the carotid sinus, which then slows the sinus. By the time of the next QRS, no further blood flow has occurred, so the sinus rate is increased. Systole then occurs, and the chain of events is repeated. If 1:1 A–V conduction resumes in such a patient, the *second*

conducted beat may manifest an increase in the P–R interval, since the last ventriculophasic vagal surge (which affects both the A–V node as well as the S–A node) is still operative. Under these circumstances, measurement of the first two P–R intervals following resumption of 1:1 conduction may erroneously suggest Mobitz I block. If the *third* beat demonstrates a *decreasing* P–R interval compared to the second, one is truly dealing with Mobitz II block (see ECG II–32). In patients with spontaneously occurring Mobitz II block, PVCs may produce infranodal delay as well as complete interruption of conduction. When such delay occurs, the beats following the PVC may also show an initial increase in the P–R interval (by up to 0.05 sec.), followed by progressive decline to baseline by the time the next spontaneous drop occurs. Here again, the mere finding of an increase in the P–R interval may lead to an erroneous diagnosis of Mobitz I block. In terms of PVC-induced Mobitz II block in general, one ordinarily expects that, given *normal* A–V conduction, a P-wave occurring within or closely following the T-wave of the PVC may not be able to conduct (because of retrograde penetration of the conducting system by the PVC). In Mobitz II block, the conduction of P-waves *remote* from the PVC is also affected (see ECGs II–21 and II–22).

Two other pitfalls in the determination of the type of 2° or advanced A–V block must be pointed out. As was previously mentioned, a vagal surge may mimic Mobitz II block; here, one looks for a slight increase in the P–R interval immediately preceding the dropped beat, as well as usually a slight increase in the P–P interval at the time of the drop. In *very long* A–V Wenckebach sequences, the P–R intervals may prolong, then remain constant for a number of beats before the drop. Therefore, when a single beat is apparently suddenly dropped, one should examine the preceding 5 to 10 beats to detect such lengthening. In addition, of course, the P–R interval of the beat following the drop would be shorter than that preceding it. (Unless the QRSs following the dropped beats have P–R intervals less than 0.12 sec., or widely varying, one can assume they are sinus captures and not junctional escapes.)

The other pitfall relates to the method of analysis. If one is dealing with advanced heart block and one finds *only two* consecutively conducted P-waves, an increase in the P–R interval between the two could be more apparent than real. This occurs when the first P–R is shorter *because it represents the fortuitous placement of a junctional escape beat shortly after a P-wave*, rather than true A–V conduc-

---

*The patient may have 2:1 A–V nodal or infra-nodal block with A–V nodal delay, or with a fixed BBB.

tion (see ECG II–33). To avoid this trap, one must first identify the junctional escape beats (review Section I, pp. 15-16). These are the QRSs which terminate the longest R–R intervals and which are unrelated to the preceding P-wave.

It must be added that, in advanced heart block, the *timing* of the P-waves relative to the escape beats may play a major role in perpetuating the block (see ECG II–35 A–C). This is particularly true in 2:1 A–V block or in an isorhythmic A–V dissociation in which the atrial rate is almost exactly double the escape rate and the QRSs maintain a nearly constant relationship to every other P-wave (pseudo-2:1). Should every other P-wave find itself near or within the T-wave of the preceding escape QRS, such P-waves would ordinarily not be expected to conduct, because of concealed penetration of the conducting system by the escape beat. The conduction pattern therefore tends to be perpetuated even if the intrinsic conductivity of the heart is relatively good.

Finally, it should be noted that a disparity often exists between antegrade and retrograde infra-nodal conduction. It is not uncommon to find 1:1 V–A conduction following implantation of a ventricular pacemaker for complete antegrade infra-nodal block. In contradistinction, when impairment of A–V nodal conduction is present, the block is usually bidirectional.

CLINICAL SIGNIFICANCE OF TYPE OF BLOCK

In advanced A–V nodal block, the escape pacemaker is located in the junctional or subjunctional (i.e., proximal bundle branch fascicles) region. Such pacemakers are usually reliable,* escaping with rates of 30 to 60/min., more so when accelerated by digitalis toxicity, acute inferior wall MI, or catecholamines. In contradistinction, in advanced infra-nodal block, the escape mechanism is located in the ventricular Purkinje system. Such idioventricular rhythms are slow, unstable, and may even completely fail to escape. Syncope ("Stokes-Adams" attacks) and death may ensue. 2° or advanced A–V nodal block may require a pacemaker if the heart rate is less than 40; if heart failure or hypotension is present; if there is serious ventricular ectopy requiring or potentially requiring antiarrhythmic therapy;** or if, in the presence of an acute inferior wall MI or digitalis toxicity, there is no response to atropine.** The patient with an

occasional Wenckebach period occurring during sleep in a non-acute setting, and who has no symptoms and no long pauses,* usually has a benign prognosis and does not require a pacemaker. (Perhaps most individuals with 1° A–V block, if monitored carefully, would be found to have an occasional A–V Wenckebach period during sleep.) On the other hand, infra-nodal block carries such a sinister prognosis that the finding of a *single dropped beat,* if by a Mobitz II mechanism, justifies immediate pacemaking. Atropine improves A–V conduction in many, but not all, patients with A–V nodal block. Atropine has no effect or may even worsen A–V conduction in patients with infra-nodal block.** While preparing to institute emergency pacemaking in such patients, an intravenous drip of isuprel may be required to establish A–V conduction if it completely or nearly completely fails. Acute bilateral BBB may complicate acute anterior wall MI.

BILEVEL A–V BLOCK

Second-degree A–V block may occur simultaneously in both the A–V node and infra-nodal system, or at two levels within the A–V node. Such bilevel 2° A–V block has been termed "alternating Wenckebach period." In A–V nodal/infra-nodal block, the underlying atrial rhythm is usually sinus with a P-wave rate of 130 bpm or less. In such cases, the A–V nodal conduction is of Wenckebach type, with additional 2:1 infra-nodal block. In bilevel A–V nodal block, the underlying atrial rate tends to be 130 bpm or more (marked sinus tachycardia, ectopic atrial tachycardia, atrial-paced rhythm, or atrial flutter). In such cases, either level has Wenckebach conduction, while the other has 2:1 block.

In all cases of bilevel 2° A–V block, nonconducted P-waves alternate with beats having progressive P–R prolongation until one of the latter also fails to conduct. When the upper level of block is Wenckebach, with 2:1 block in the lower level (i.e., A–V nodal/infra-nodal or A–V nodal/A–V nodal), a total of *two* nonconducted P-waves occur during the pause. These two P-waves represent the fixed 2:1 dropped beat plus the Wenckebach dropped beat. Following the pause created by the Wenckebach dropped beat, conduction in the lower level has had the opportunity to recover, so the following P-wave conducts; the expected 2:1 dropped beat does not occur (see Figure II–2).

---

*One prominent exception is severe hypothyroidism, where the escape mechanisms may be suppressed (see ECG II–16).
**Antiarrhythmic agents may suppress subsidiary escape pacemakers or surround them with "exit block."

*A minimum of 3.0 sec. is required for "pre-syncope," 5.0 sec. for syncope.
**Also, antiarrhythmic agents and hyperkalemia exacerbate infra-nodal block.

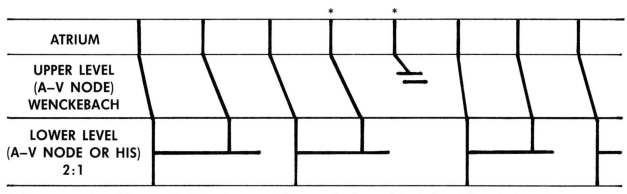

A. Two nonconducted P-waves (*) during the pause. The upper level Wenckebach drop *follows* the lower level 2:1 drop.

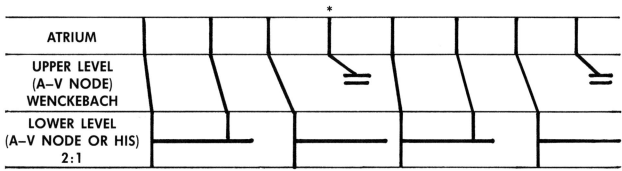

B. One nonconducted P-wave (*) alternates with each conducted beat. The upper level Wenckebach drop *coincides* with the lower level 2:1 drop.

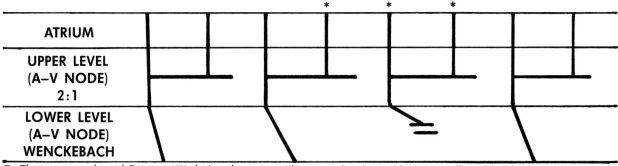

C. Three nonconducted P-waves (*) during the pause. The upper level 2:1 block is unaffected by the lower level delay.

Figure II–2. Bilevel 2° A–V block ("alternating Wenckebach periods").

When the upper level of block is 2:1, with Wenckebach conduction in the lower level (i.e., A–V nodal/A–V nodal), a total of *three* nonconducted P-waves occur during the pause. These three P-waves represent the fixed 2:1 dropped beat, followed by the Wenckebach dropped beat, *followed in turn by the next fixed 2:1 dropped beat.*

Since the pause produced by the Wenckebach drop occurs in the lower level, no delay of the next beat's presentation to the upper level is incurred (see Figure II–2).

The above two- and three-P-wave rules apply with three exceptions: (1) in bilevel 2° A–V block alternating with simple A–V nodal Wenckebach

TABLE II–3. A–V Block.

I. A–V nodal
   A. Simple
      1. 1° (P–R of 0.21 to 0.60 sec.)
      2. 2° (A–V Wenckebach periods, Mobitz Type I)
      3. Advanced (including "complete")
   B. Complex (bi-level)
      *1. Sinus tachycardia or ectopic atrial tachycardia with Wenckebach upper nodal plus 2:1 lower nodal
      2. Atrial flutter with:
         **a. "3:1 conduction" (3:2 Wenckebach upper nodal plus 2:1 lower nodal)
         #b. "Alternating 2:1/4:1" (2:1 upper nodal plus 3:2 Wenckebach lower nodal)
      3. Various rhythms (sinus, atrial fibrillation, etc.) with complete block in the upper node and reentry in the lower node.
II. Infra-nodal (His bundle or bilateral BBB)
   A. 1° (delay of 0.05 sec. or less)
   B. 2°
      1. Mobitz Type II (sinus rhythm)
      (2. Wenckebach conduction in a single bundle branch)
   C. Advanced (including "complete")
III. Combined A–V nodal and Infra-nodal
   A. 1° A–V nodal plus 2° (Mobitz Type II) or advanced infra-nodal
   *B. 2° A–V nodal plus 2:1 infra-nodal
   C. 3° A–V nodal plus 2° infra-nodal (accelerated junctional rhythm with H–V Wenckebach periods)

*"Alternating Wenckebach period" with 1 or 2 dropped beats during pause.
**The lower level of block may, in some instances, be located in the His bundle. In such cases, the block is functional, that is, produced by "long-short" H–H cycles created by the 3:2 block in the A–V node.
#"Alternating Wenckebach period" with three dropped beats during pause.

periods; (2) as a result of the "gap phenomenon," when, following a large increase in A–V nodal (A–H) delay, the concomitant H–H interval is sufficiently increased to allow conduction of the His-Purkinje system to recover by the time the impulse is presented to it; and (3) when the 2:1 lower level drop *coincides with* the Wenckebach drop on the upper level (in the usual case they do not coincide—see Figure II–2). In all three exceptions, the expected number of nonconducted P-waves during the pause is reduced by one.

Other degrees of bilevel conduction abnormalities also occur. First-degree A–V nodal block may be combined with 2° or advanced infra-nodal block. Complete A–V nodal block may be combined with accelerated junctional rhythm and H–V Wenckebach periods. Finally, there may rarely occur a situation in which there is complete A–V dissociation between an A–V nodal reentry loop (or sustained reentrant SVT) and either sinus rhythm or AF; under these circumstances, there is

complete A–V nodal block restricted only to the upper reaches of the node (see ECG II–44).

A classification of the various types of A–V block is summarized in Table II–3.

BRADYARRHYTHMIAS RELATED TO SINUS FUNCTION

The various bradyarrhythmias related to sinus function are summarized in Table II–4. Long pauses may occur with sustained *marked sinus bradycardia* (rate less than 40/min.). *Sinus arrest* produces a long asystolic pause (> 2.0 sec.) which is *not a multiple* of the basic sinus rate. The mechanism is the failure of the S–A node to depolarize. Such a long pause may be terminated by a sinus beat, or atrial, junctional, or ventricular escape beat. Severe depression (> 3.0 sec.) of the S–A node may also occur after any of the various atrial tachyarrhythmias or following a single PAC; again the sinus, atrium, junction or ventricle may escape. In many cases of such "tachy-brady syndromes," the sinus beats immediately subsequent to the first sinus escape may yield long secondary pauses. Finally, severe S–A block (also called Type II S–A block) may occur. Here the long asystolic pause is equal to *a precise multiple* of the basic sinus rate; the mechanism is the failure of one or more sinus depolarizations to break out of the S–A node into the surrounding atrium. Any or all of these bradyarrhythmias may constitute a "sick sinus syndrome" in a given individual. Production of the long pauses in all the above depends not only upon the presence of a "sick sinus," but also upon a diseased junctional escape mechanism. "Sick sinus syndromes" may be produced or exacerbated by Type I antiarrhythmic agents (therapeutic and

TABLE II–4. Bradyarrhythmias Related to Sinus Function.

I. Sinus bradycardia
   A. Mild (40–60 bpm)
   *B. Severe (< 40 bpm)
II. Sinus node depression (spontaneous)
   A. Mild (sinus pause, < 2.0 sec.)
   *B. Severe (sinus arrest, > 2.0 sec.)
III. Sinus node depression (post-PAC, PAT, atrial fibrillation or flutter)
   A. Mild (< 3.0 sec., normally seen; subsequent sinus beats show adequate rate)
   *B. Severe (> 3.0 sec.; "tachy-brady syndrome;" subsequent sinus beats often show secondary long pauses)
IV. S–A block
   A. Mild (S–A Wenckebach periods, Type I)
   *B. Severe (2:1 or more advanced S–A block, Type II)

*Any or all may constitute a "sick sinus syndrome."

toxic doses), by propranolol, by digitalis intoxication, or as an idiosyncratic reaction to digitalis or Aldomet. *Therapeutic* doses of digitalis usually do not worsen sinus function, even if already impaired. Occasionally a "sick sinus syndrome" presents itself as an atrial tachyarrhythmia (AF, atrial flutter, PAT) *with a slow heart rate in the absence of digitalis.**

Mild versions of the serious sinus bradyarrhythmias may occur. These include mild sinus bradycardia (40 to 60/min.); spontaneous sinus pauses (sinus "arrest" of under 2.0 sec.); mild suppression of the *first* sinus beat post-PAC (PAT, or other atrial tachyarrhythmia)—in such cases, the pause is usually under 3.0 sec. and subsequent sinus beats occur at a reasonable rate; and S–A block of Wenckebach type (Type I S–A block). Although all may occur in normal individuals, S–A Wenckebach block may result from vagotonic drugs and maneuvers, as well as from digitalis intoxication. In S–A Wenckebach periods, "group beating" of the QRSs

is related to "group beating" of the P-waves; the P–P intervals progressively shorten before the pause.* Many patients with digitalis-toxicity-induced S–A Wenckebach periods have concurrent A–V Wenckebach periods. In such patients, the P–R intervals progressively increase as the P–P intervals progressively decrease. A dropped QRS occurs only if the length of the S–A Wenckebach period exceeds that of the A–V Wenckebach period.

BRADYARRHYTHMIAS RELATED TO MASSIVE VAGAL SURGE

During massive vagal surges there is profound slowing of the sinus as well as A–V block. Vasovagal attacks, protracted vomiting, or carotid sinus hypersensitivity are the usual causes. The first two acutely respond to fluids and atropine; a permanent pacemaker may be required for the latter.

---

*DC shock may result in a flatline.

*The sinus-to-atrium (or S–A) intervals, which cannot be measured on the ECG, progressively lengthen.

SECTION II
Electrocardiograms

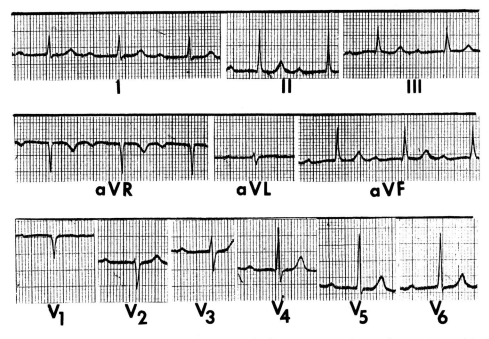

ECG II–1. *Sinus rhythm with first-degree A–V block.* The heart rate is 67 bpm. The P–R interval is 0.40 sec.

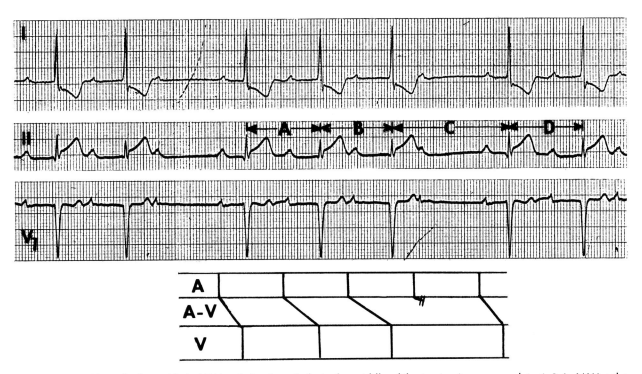

ECG II–2. *Sinus rhythm with A–V Wenckebach periods.* In the middle of the tracing is one complete 4:3 A–V Wenckebach period. The sinus rate is 70 bpm. A–V conduction time, represented by the P–R interval, progressively increases until one beat is finally dropped. This is a typical A–V Wenckebach period. The R–R intervals decrease as the P–R intervals increase (i.e., cycle A > cycle B). The length of the pause containing the dropped beat is less than that of the two previous cycles (i.e., C < A + B); it is also less than twice the length of the previous cycle (i.e., C < 2 × B). The length of the cycle following the pause is greater than that preceding it (i.e., D > B).* In this case there are 4 P-waves producing 3 QRSs, hence, a 4:3 A–V Wenckebach period. The Wenckebach nature of the A–V conduction indicates the site of block is in the A–V node. In the case of this patient, the block was caused by an acute inferior wall myocardial infarction.

A = Atria; A–V = A–V Node; V = Ventricles.

*This is, of course, not true of a 3:2 A–V Wenckebach period.

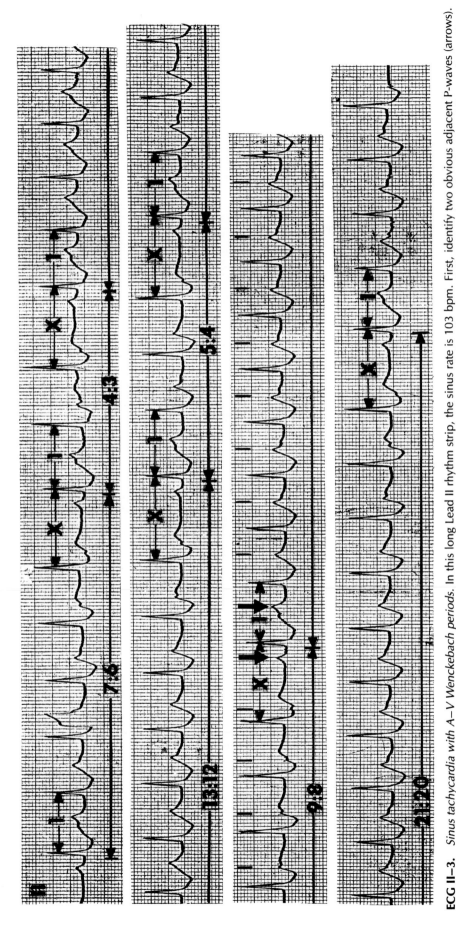

ECG II-3. *Sinus tachycardia with A–V Wenckebach periods.* In this long Lead II rhythm strip, the sinus rate is 103 bpm. First, identify two obvious adjacent P-waves (arrows). Then continue measuring one P–P cycle in either direction. The calipers fall upon each P-wave, enabling rapid identification of all P-waves buried in the ST and T complexes. Next, notice the relatively long R–R intervals (X), and observe the nonconducted P-wave contained in each. Finally, sequentially measure the P–R intervals belonging to the cluster of beats contained between these larger R–R intervals. Progressive P–R prolongation culminating in the dropped beat is consistently observed. Observe the noticeable "group beating" effect created by the mild but definite decrease of the R–R intervals in each of the smaller clusters of beats; in each case, the first R–R interval (1) is the longest within the cluster, since the greatest increment of A–V nodal delay occurs at the beginning of the A–V Wenckebach period (i.e., typical Wenckebach period). In this ECG, some of the A–V Wenckebach periods are quite long. In the 21:20 cluster, observe that beyond the first three beats, beat-to-beat changes in the P–R and R–R intervals are minimal. The dropped beat at the end of such a long sequence could be mistaken for a sudden dropped beat (i.e., for infra-nodal, Mobitz II block). In this patient, the cause of the A–V block was digitalis toxicity.

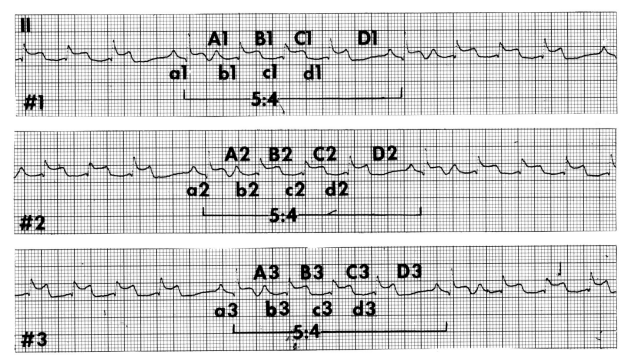

ECG II–4.   *Sinus tachycardia with A–V Wenckebach periods.* These are typical A–V Wenckebach periods, producing a "group-beating" effect. Notice how precise is the replication of Wenckebach sequences having the same ratio. In this ECG, the homologous P–Rs and R–Rs within each 5:4 sequence are identical, as are therefore the lengths of the entire sequence.* Note the acute inferior wall MI (Lead II).

---

*The length of 5:4 cycle #1 = #2 = #3. Within each cycle, A1 = A2 = A3, a1 = a2 = a3, etc.

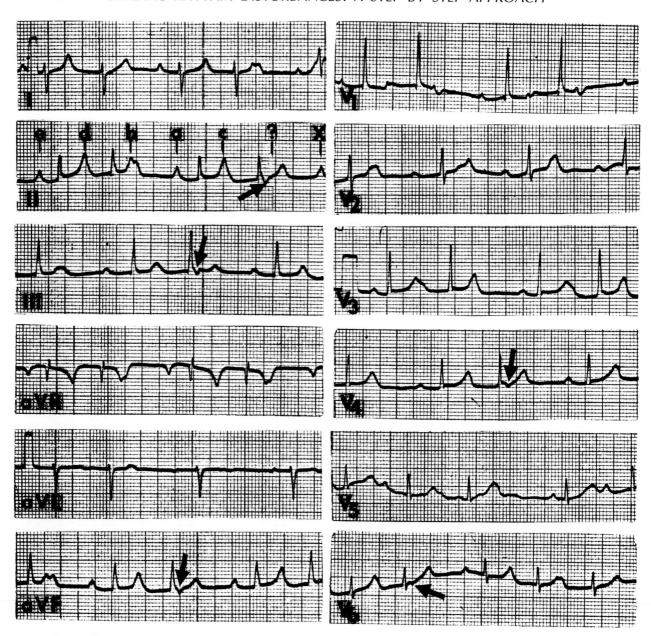

ECG II–5. *A–V Wenckebach periods, some of which are terminated by atrial echoes.* Examine Lead II. One P-wave (a) in the middle of the strip is obviously identifiable. The preceding T-wave has an obvious deformity (b); the following T-wave is tall and peaked (c). By setting one's calipers on a and b, one finds that cycle ab = cycle ac. By continuing to measure back, P-waves d and e fall into place. Once these sinus-P-waves (rate 110 bpm) have been identified, it is evident that Lead II begins with a 3:2 A–V Wenckebach period. After the dropped beat, another A–V Wenckebach sequence begins. However, the second QRS of this sequence seems to have an "S-wave" (arrow). It is conceivable that this QRS could be a RBBB by virtue of functional aberration (i.e., because of the "long-short" cycle sequence caused by the pause containing the dropped beat). However, careful analysis reveals this not to be the case. Note that the next sinus-P-wave after C should have occurred in the place indicated by the question mark—but it did not. Instead, the next sinus-P-wave (X) *seems to be reset one cycle from the "S-wave"* (reset time equals one sinus P–P cycle plus the usual 100 or so msec. increment). It is now clear that the arrow points not to an S-wave but to a *retrograde-P-wave, representing an atrial echo.* Because c conducts so slowly through the A–V node, by the time it reaches the lower part of the node it finds another pathway within the node whose conduction has sufficiently recovered to permit retrograde conduction back to the atria. Why did c result in an atrial echo and d did not? The P–R interval following c is longer than that following d. Presumably, all the pathways within the A–V node were still refractory when d reached the lower portion of the node. (Even if the P–R intervals had measured to be the same, a difference of several msec., perhaps crucial for reentry, is not measurable on the ECG; even if truly identical, the refractoriness of the A–V node might have been slightly different owing to changes of autonomic tone, etc.)

The atrial echoes in other leads are also identified (arrows). Note the striking RVH pattern of the QRSs. The patient was a young adult with Tetralogy of Fallot.

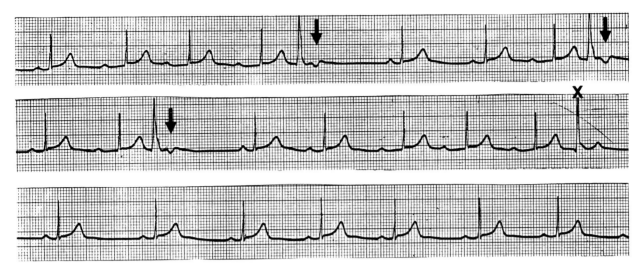

ECG II–6. *A–V Wenckebach periods terminated by PVCs.* There is mild sinus arrhythmia. In one case (X) the PVC renders the conducting system refractory because of concealed retrograde conduction in the A–V node. The other three PVCs terminate the A–V Wenckebach periods by conducting retrogradely to the atria to produce retrograde-P-waves (arrows).

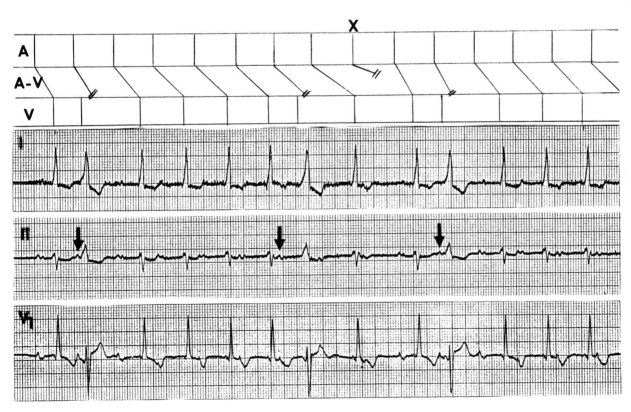

ECG II–7. *A–V Wenckebach periods with PVCs.* The sinus rate is 97 bpm. The three early, bizarre, and wider QRSs are PVCs. Ignoring the PVCs, one notices two sequences during which the P–R intervals progressively increase. In each case, the P–R interval of the beat following the PVC is longer than the P–R interval of the beat preceding it. This indicates that the PVCs do not interrupt A–V conduction, and that the three P-waves (arrows) immediately preceding the PVCs do not produce QRSs because of simple preemption of the ventricles by the PVCs. Thus, the only true dropped beat (X) terminates one 9:8 A–V Wenckebach period and heralds another (at least 6:5). Although disruptive to the eye, the PVCs do not interrupt the basic A–V Wenckebach sequences.

A = Atria; A–V = A–V Node; V = Ventricles.

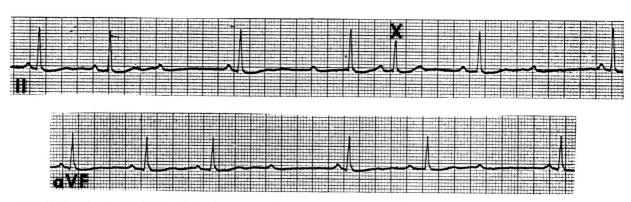

ECG II–8. *Atypical A–V Wenckebach period in the presence of sinus arrhythmia.* Lead II begins with an apparent 3:2 A–V Wenckebach sequence. Following the dropped beat, the P–R interval markedly increases, then decreases, then slightly increases before the next dropped beat.* Note the significant sinus arrhythmia at the time of the fluctuating P–R intervals. At other times, as well as in Lead aVF, when the sinus rate is less erratic, A–V conduction is that of typical A–V Wenckebach periods. Presumably, during the period of significant sinus arrhythmia, changes in both the P–P and P–R intervals reflect fluctuating autonomic tone. The atypical A–V Wenckebach period is thus diagnosed by both the noticeable increase of the P–R interval several beats before the drop, as well as by the "company it keeps," that is, by the presence of obvious, typical A–V Wenckebach periods.

---

*It is assumed that X is not a fortuitously occurring PJC, or a ventricular echo from an abortive atrial echo (see ECG II–35 C). Presumably, the beat is conducted with mild functional aberration because of the "long-short" cycle relationship.

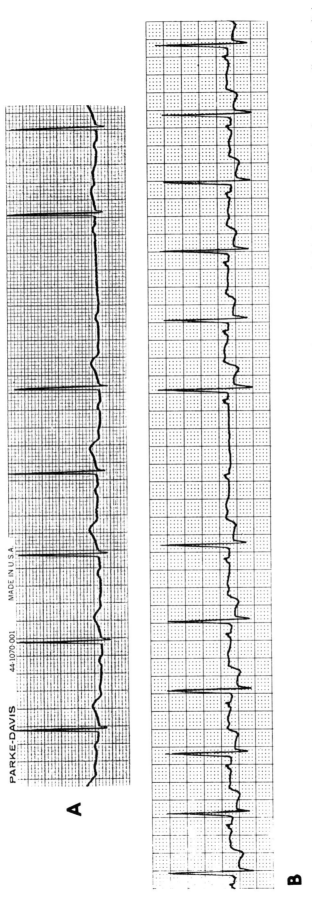

ECG II–9. A and B. *Atypical A–V Wenckebach periods due to "vagal surge."* Note the slight increase in the P–R interval of the beat preceding the drop, as well as the slight increase of the P–P interval around the time of the drop. Such vagal surges commonly occur during sleep.

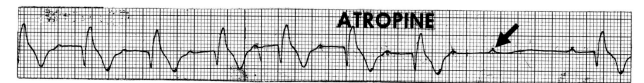

ECG II–10. *Atypical A–V Wenckebach period with two nonconducted P-waves.* Following slight progressive P–R prolongation, a dropped beat occurs. Presumably, this is the end of a long A–V Wenckebach period, during which beat-to-beat P–R interval changes may be minor (or even constant for a number of beats). Following the nonconducted sinus-P-wave, a second, early, nonconducted P-wave (arrow) occurs. This nonconducted PAC then resets the sinus. Presumably, the nonconducted sinus-P-wave penetrated enough of the A–V node to render that tissue refractory to the early PAC, so that it, too, failed to conduct.

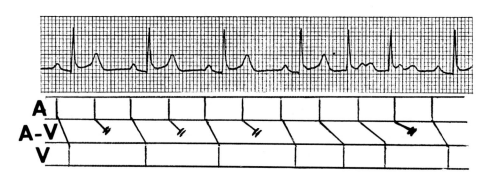

ECG II–11. *A–V Wenckebach period unmasking 2:1 A–V conduction.* Although the rhythm at first appears to be sinus, there are two "early beats," which are interspersed with "extra" P-waves. However, one quickly notices that the T-waves of these two beats are not as tall as the "control" T-waves, and, in fact, represent the pure T-waves. The sinus rate is double the apparent sinus rate at the beginning of the rhythm strip; the nonconducted P-waves sit almost perfectly atop the apex of the T-waves. The "early" beats actually represent improvement of A–V conduction from 2:1 to 4:3 Wenckebach. Even if the 2:1 block had been immediately recognized, the presence of the A–V Wenckebach period also pinpoints the site of block to the A–V node.

A = Atria; A–V = A–V Node; V = Ventricles.

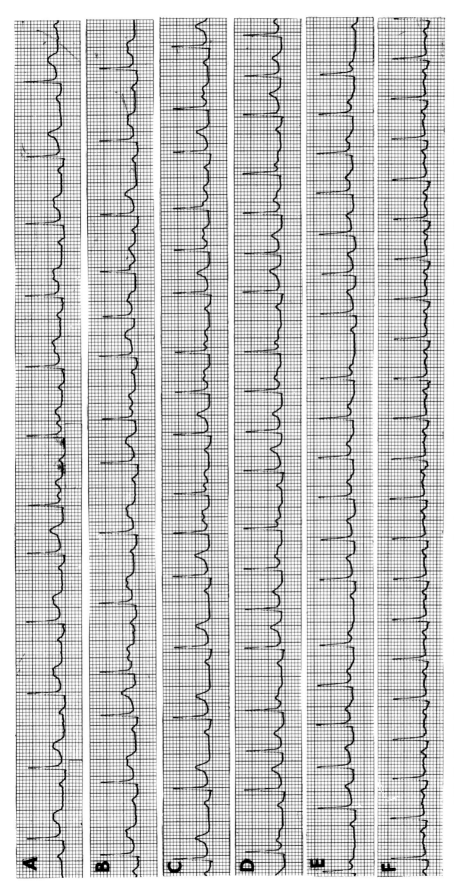

ECG II–12. *Strips A through F represent progressive improvement of A–V (nodal) conduction in a patient with an acute inferior wall M.I.*

A. 2:1 A–V conduction; one 3:2 A–V Wenckebach period.
B. 2:1, 3:2, 4:3 A–V conduction.
C. 2:1, 4:3, 3:2 A–V conduction.
D. 4:3, 5:4 A–V Wenckebach periods.
E. 6:5, 7:6, 8:7 A–V Wenckebach periods.
F. 1:1 A–V conduction.

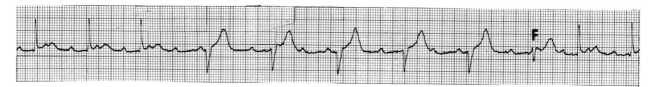

ECG II–13.   *Same patient as shown in II–12.* 2:1 A–V block with a period of advanced ("complete") heart block. During this period there is A–V dissociation with a subjunctional or ventricular escape rhythm which emerges at 56 bpm, then "warms up" slightly to 58 bpm. A–V conduction then resumes. "F" represents a fusion between the escape pacemaker and a conducted beat. From this rhythm strip alone, the site of A–V block cannot be ascertained. However, in the setting of an acute inferior wall M.I., as well as with the subsequent improvement of A–V conduction manifested by A–V Wenckebach periods (see II–12), the A–V node can be inferred as the site of block.

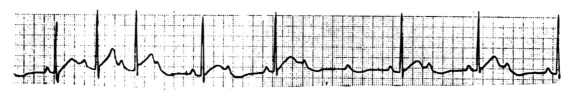

ECG II–14.   *Advanced A–V block in the A–V node.* Following a 4:3 A–V Wenckebach period, A–V conduction decreases to 2:1, then 3:1, then returns to 2:1. That the A–V node is the site of the advanced block is inferred by the "company it keeps," namely, the A–V Wenckebach period.

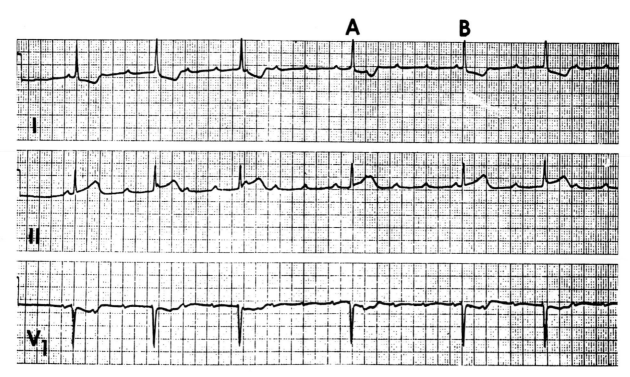

ECG II–15.   *Advanced A–V block during acute inferior wall M.I.* In this clinical context, the site of block is the A–V node. However, without this information, the site of block cannot be ascertained from the rhythm alone, since there are no two consecutively conducted P-waves. A and B represent junctional escape beats, since they terminate the longest (and equal) R–R intervals, and have no relationship to their respective preceding P-wave. The other QRSs presumably represent conducted beats.

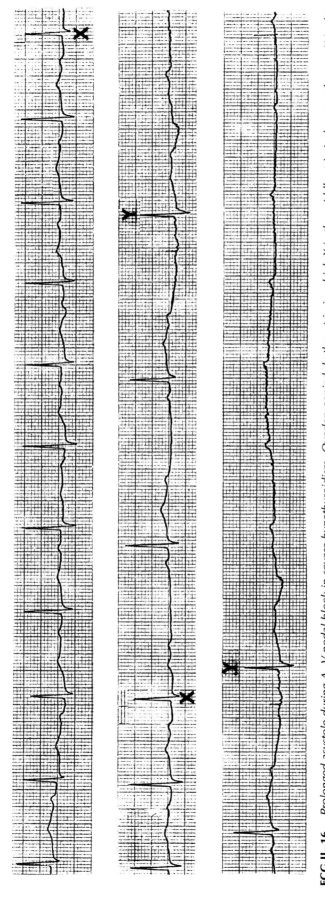

ECG II–16. *Prolonged asystole during A–V nodal block in severe hypothyroidism. Overlap-copied rhythm strip in which X in the middle strip is the same beat as X in the top strip; the two Ys also label the same beat. Following a long A–V Wenckebach period, there is a decrease in A–V conduction to 2:1 followed by a prolonged period of complete heart block without any escape beats. Such prolonged asystolic periods are much more characteristic of advanced infra-nodal block than of advanced A–V nodal block. In this case, however, the A–V Wenckebach period localizes the site of block to the A–V node. The lack of an adequate escape mechanism was presumably the result of the patient's markedly hypothyroid state.*

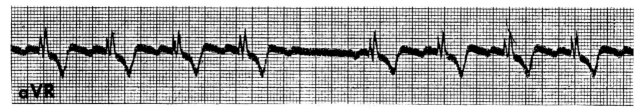

ECG II–17. *Mobitz II A–V block.* There is a sudden dropped beat. All the P–R intervals are identical. RBBB is present; presumably, the drop occurred because of sudden bilateral bundle branch block.

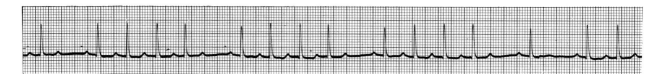

ECG II–18. *Mobitz II A–V block.* There are sudden dropped beats; the P–R intervals are unchanging. Interestingly, one nonconducted PAC is also present. Can you find it? The QRS-complexes are narrow; presumably, the site of block is the bundle of His.

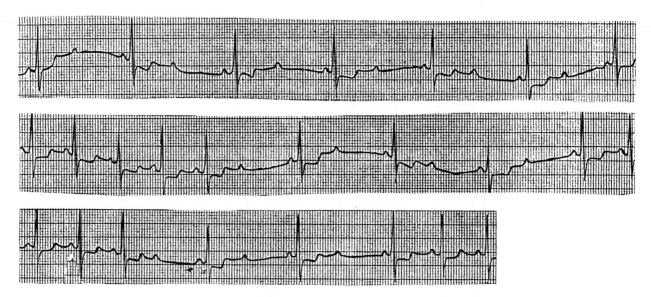

ECG II–19. *Advanced infra-nodal block.* There are periods of 2:1 A–V block. The P–R intervals of consecutively conducted beats demonstrate no change.

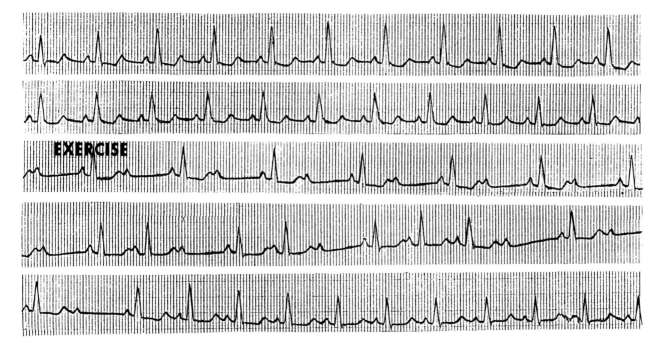

ECG II–20. *Mobitz II second-degree and advanced infra-nodal block precipitated by exercise.* Sporadic single dropped beats (Mobitz II) as well as periods of 2:1 A–V block occur. The P–R intervals of the consecutively conducted beats are unchanging, indicating infra-nodal block.

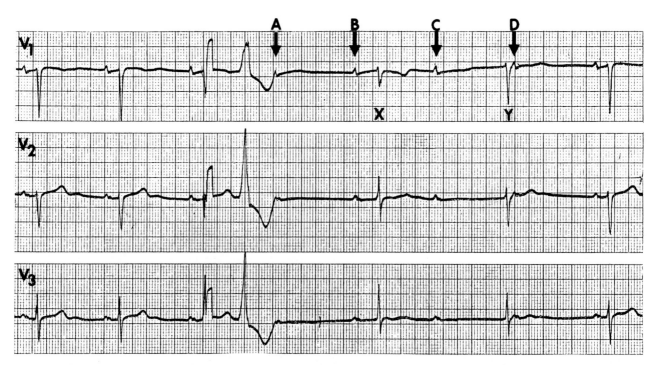

ECG II–21. *Advanced infra-nodal block precipitated by a PVC.* There are three beats of sinus rhythm, the third of which is in "fusion" with the ECG standardization mark. The sinus-P-wave immediately following the PVC (A) is too close to the T-wave to be expected to conduct. However, there follows a period of A–V dissociation during which a slow escape rhythm, consisting of two beats (X and Y), emerges. The cause of the A–V dissociation is advanced ("complete") heart block, since P-waves B and C should have been able to conduct. That B is nonconducted is strongly inferred from four observations: (1) the P–R interval following B is longer than the P–Rs of the three conducted beats, (2) C clearly does not conduct, (3) the morphology of the QRS following B varies somewhat from that of the first three beats, (4) the interval between the end of the PVC and X is approximately the same as that between X and Y; since Y is unquestionably an escape beat, X probably is, too. X and Y differ slightly in morphology, presumably because they originate from two slightly different fascicular locations. Following D, which is too close to Y to be able to conduct, even if intrinsically capable of doing so, A–V conduction resumes. To summarize, advanced heart block precipitated by a PVC is present. This type of presentation indicates the site of block is almost certainly infra-nodal. (Reproduced with permission from Childers, R.: Classification of cardiac dysrhythmias. Med. Clin. North Am., *60:3,* 1976.)

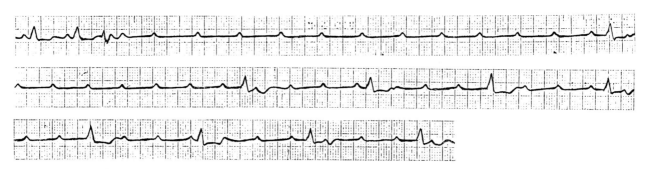

ECG II–22. *Advanced infra-nodal block precipitated by a PVC.* As in II–21, advanced A–V block follows the PVC. In this case, however, the block is prolonged and the escape mechanism is inadequate. (Reproduced with permission from Childers, R.: Classification of cardiac dysrhythmias. Med. Clin. North Am., *60:3,* 1976.)

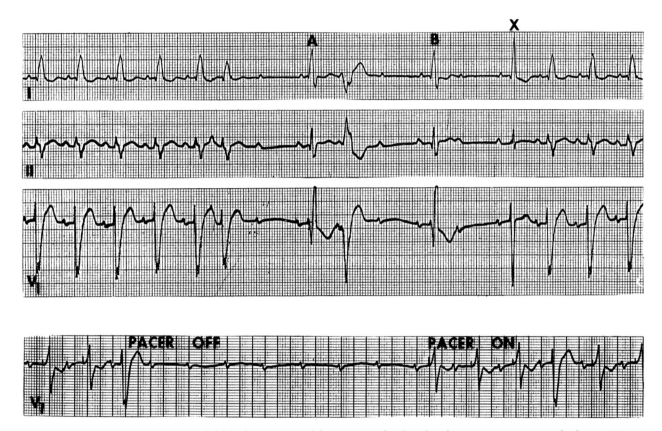

ECG II–23. *Advanced infra-nodal block precipitated by a PAC.* The first five beats represent sinus rhythm. LBBB is present. Following a PAC, there is a period of advanced A–V block, during which there are two escape beats (A and B) arising from or near the left bundle. (Note the lack of constancy of the P–R interval preceding these beats.) One PVC is also present. As sinus rhythm resumes, the first beat (X) occurs with a narrow QRS and a longer than normal P–R interval. This beat represents a conducted beat *with bilateral bundle branch delay,* and indicates that conduction is at times possible in the left bundle.* The development of advanced A–V block following a PAC indicates infra-nodal block. It is, of course, not known whether the block in this example represents His bundle block or bilateral bundle branch block. A pacemaker was inserted. The bottom strip illustrates two important points: (1) The spontaneous occurrence of advanced A–V block in patients in whom the block is precipitated by an extrasystole, and, (2) the unreliability or the escape mechanism in infra-nodal block.

---

*A fusion between a conducted and escape beat would have produced a narrow QRS, but with a *shorter than normal* P–R interval.

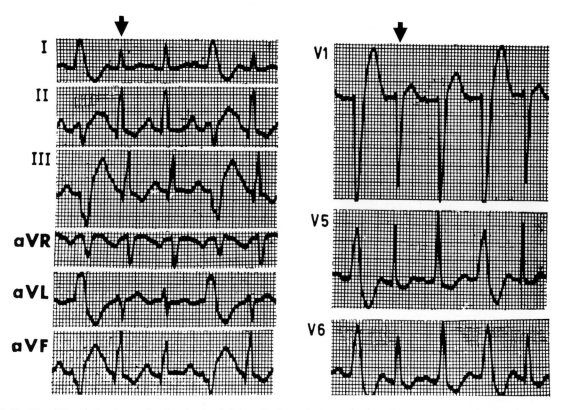

ECG II–24. *Wenckebach conduction in the left bundle branch.* In each three-beat sequence, the first beat (arrow) is conducted normally. The second beat is conducted with incomplete LBBB, the third beat with complete LBBB. The sequence then resumes. Left bundle conduction can therefore be characterized as 3:2 Wenckebach type. The third beat, showing complete LBBB, represents the dropped beat in the left bundle. Although the conduction is of Wenckebach type, it indicates severe disease of the left bundle; should RBBB develop, complete bilateral bundle branch block could occur (see II–25). (Reproduced with permission from Friedberg, H. D., and Schamroth, L.: The Wenckebach phenomenon in left bundle branch block. Am. J. Cardiol., *24*:591, 1969.)

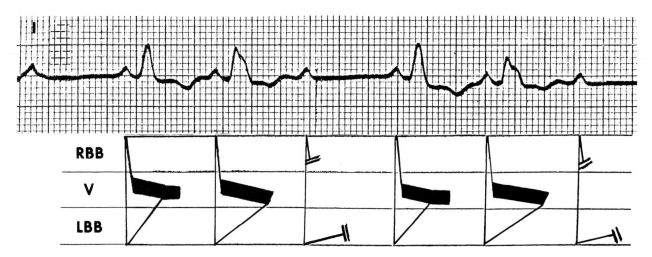

ECG II–25. *3:2 Wenckebach conduction in the left bundle branch with coexisting 3:2 Mobitz II block in the right bundle branch.* The first beat is conducted with incomplete LBBB. The second beat is conducted with complete LBBB; conduction in the left bundle could be absent, but may merely be too slow to reach the left ventricle before it is activated by the impulse exiting from the right bundle. A third beat is dropped. There is no conduction in either the right or left bundle. Again, the Wenckebach conduction in the left bundle bespeaks severe disease. Prolonged periods of asystole could develop in this patient.

RBB = Right Bundle Branch; V = Ventricles; LBB = Left Bundle Branch.

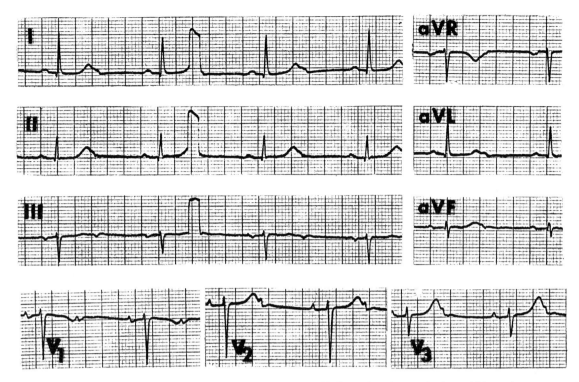

ECG II–26. *Fixed 2:1 A–V block.* The second P-wave is partially buried in the T. Block could be either A–V nodal or infra-nodal. Two consecutively conducted P-waves are required to make the differentiation.

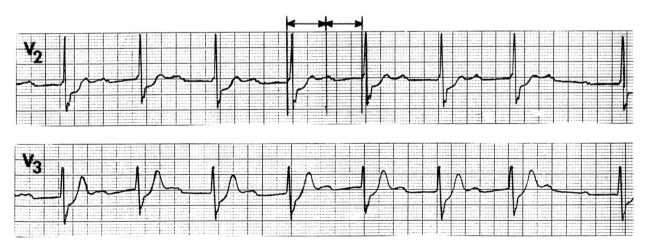

ECG II–27. *Fixed 2:1, 3:1 A–V block.* The initial deflection of the second P-wave is inscribed just before the onset of the QRS. When A–V conduction spontaneously decreases to 3:1, the true P-wave rate becomes obvious. If this had not occurred, and one had not made the measurement indicated on the ECG, the rhythm would have been erroneously diagnosed as sinus with first-degree A–V block. As in II–26, the site of the block cannot be ascertained. That the P–R interval is long does not aid in this differentiation.

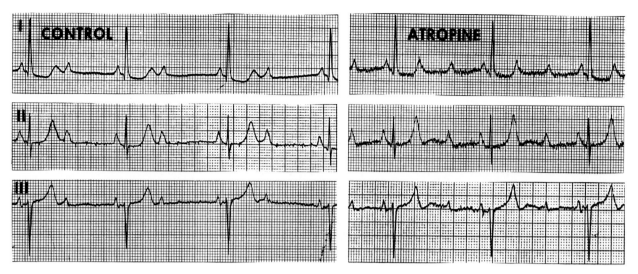

ECG II–28. *Response to atropine in fixed 2:1 A–V block.* In fixed 2:1 or more advanced A–V block, the administration of atropine is potentially dangerous, unless the clinical circumstances of digitalis toxicity or acute inferior wall MI point to the A–V node as the site of block. If the block is infra-nodal, atropine, by increasing the sinus rate, may *worsen* the degree of block. In this case, for example, the block increased from 2:1 to 3:1.

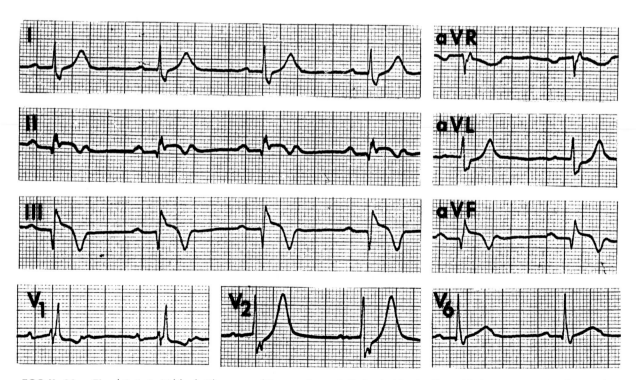

ECG II–29. *Fixed 2:1 A–V block.* The *second* P-wave is partially buried in the T, and is best seen in Leads II and V₁. Although RBBB is present, the patient clearly has an acute inferodorsal MI. The site of block is almost certainly the A–V node.

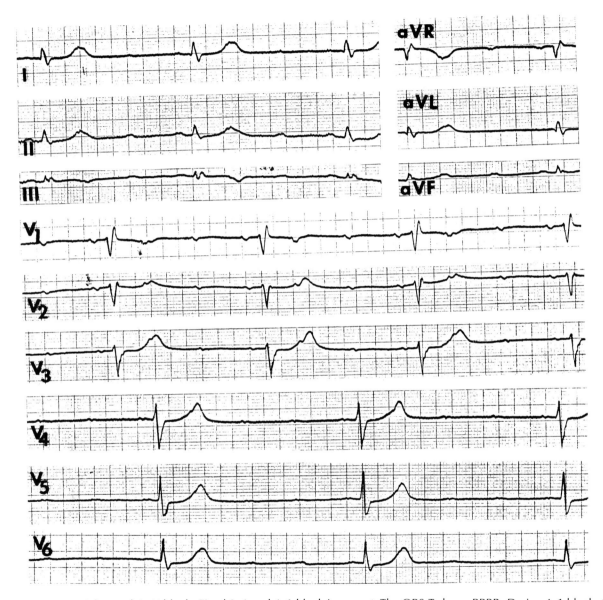

ECG II–30. *Advanced A–V block. Fixed 3:1 and 4:1 block is present.* The QRS-T shows RBBB. During 4:1 block, the heart rate is 23 bpm. The site of block could be either the A–V node or the His-Purkinje system. The latter, particularly bilateral bundle branch block, is more likely on the basis of the slow heart rate without an adequate escape rhythm.

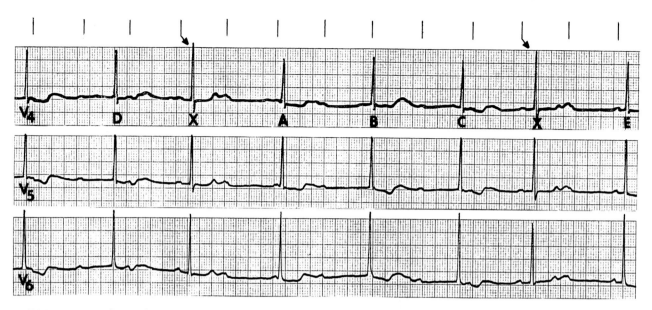

ECG II–31.   *Advanced A–V block with periods of junctional rhythm.* The sinus rate is 80 bpm. The heart rate is slow and irregular, with many obviously nonconducted P-waves. In the middle of the rhythm strip, there is an obvious period of A–V dissociation. Closer examination of beats A, B, and C reveals a junctional escape rhythm which slightly "warms up" from 40 to 43 bpm. Beats D and E terminate similar R–R intervals and are preceded by grossly different "P–R intervals"; they, too, are junctional escape beats. Beats X terminate shorter R–R intervals and are, therefore, captures. In fact, both beats are preceded by P–R intervals of equal length. Since only two captures, which are nonconsecutive, are present, the site of block cannot be determined. There is advanced A–V block, incomplete A–V dissociation with periods of junctional rhythm.

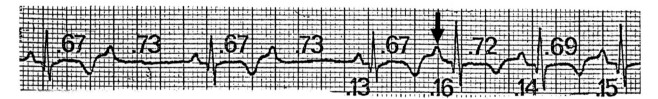

ECG II–32.   *Resumption of 1:1 conduction after 2:1 A–V block with ventriculophasic effect.* During 2:1 block, there is a ventriculophasic effect in which the P–P intervals surrounding each QRS are shorter than those between the QRSs. The P–P intervals are indicated on the ECG. It must be remembered that the carotid sinus reflex, responsible for slowing the sinus rate after the inscription of the nonconducted P-wave, also slows conduction in the A–V node. During 2:1 A–V block, since the second P-wave is nonconducted, this effect cannot be seen. Upon resumption of 1:1 conduction, the second P-wave (arrow), previously nonconducted, can now conduct. The vagally mediated effect on A–V conduction may become manifest. In this case, the P–R interval indeed shows a transient increase. As 1:1 conduction continues, the ventriculophasic effect disappears, and the P–R intervals decrease to baseline. If the above is not kept in mind, examination of the first two P–R intervals after resumption of 1:1 A–V conduction may lead to the erroneous conclusion of Wenckebach conduction, and, therefore, the A–V node as the site of block. In fact, from the information presented in this rhythm strip, the site of the block cannot be ascertained.

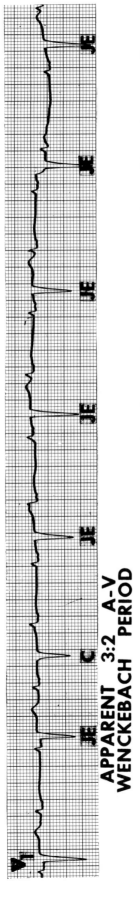

APPARENT 3:2 A-V WENCKEBACH PERIOD

ECG II-33. *Advanced A–V block.* The heart rate is slow. Many of the P-waves are obviously nonconducted. Six beats terminate long R–R intervals corresponding to rates of between 40 and 42 bpm. Since the P–R intervals preceding these beats vary, they are therefore junctional escape beats (JE). A single capture (C) terminates the one shorter R–R interval in the rhythm strip. There is therefore advanced A–V block with incomplete A–V dissociation. Because no two consecutively conducted P-waves are present, the site of block cannot be ascertained. If the junctional escape beats had not been identified first, and one merely "eyeballed" the ECG, one might reach the erroneous conclusion that the A–V node was the site of block, based on the observation of an apparent 3:2 A–V Wenckebach period. The step-by-step analysis, however, reveals that C is the only capture. As a point of added interest, note the ventriculophasic effect developed toward the end of the rhythm strip. Although A–V dissociation is present, the timing of the QRSs relative to the P-waves, the 2:1 ratio of Ps to QRSs, and the slow heart rate all combine to produce it.

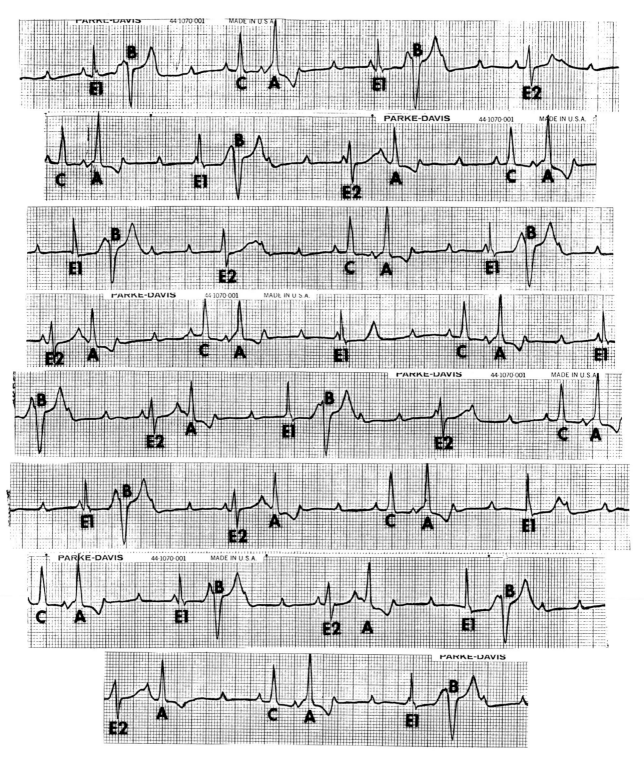

ECG II–34. *Advanced A–V block with captures, escape beats, and PVCs.* On initial inspection of the rhythm strips, two facts become obvious: (1) there is advanced heart block, with many nonconducted P-waves, and, (2) there are a number of different QRS morphologies. There are three populations of late QRSs (terminating long R–R intervals). The sinus captures (C) have uniform (R) morphology and preceding P–R interval. Escape beats E1 all have qRs morphology, follow the early upright beats (A) by a nearly constant interval, and are unrelated to their preceding P-wave. Escape beats E2 all have RS morphology, follow the early negative beats (B) by their own constant interval, and are also dissociated from the P-waves. The early, wide, bizarre, upright (A) and negative (B) beats are PVCs. Interestingly, PVC-B beats, by virtue of their site of origin or intramyocardial conduction pattern, are able to suppress E1, permitting E2 to escape. There is advanced heart block, but without two consecutively conducted P-waves, the site of block cannot be ascertained.

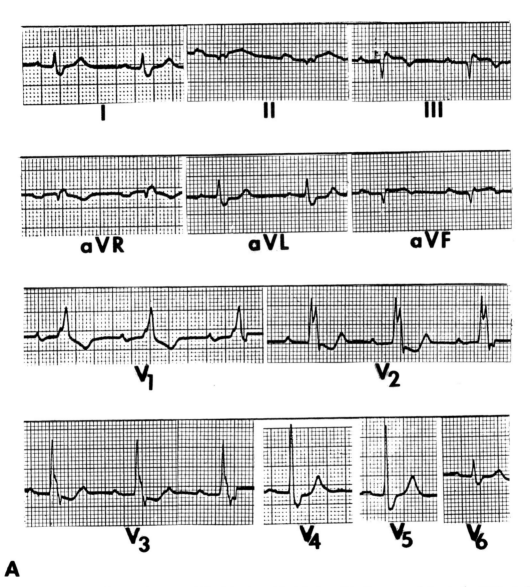

A

ECG II–35. *Perpetuation of "complete" A–V block by the critical timing of the P-waves relative to the QRSs. A. Baseline 12-lead ECG shows SR with first-degree A–V block, complete RBBB, and an (acute) inferior wall MI.*

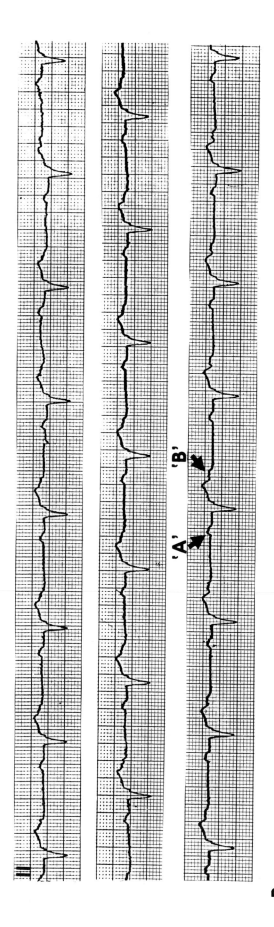

ECG II-35 (cont'd).   B. Continuous Lead II rhythm strip taken several hours later reveals "complete" heart block with a subjunctional escape rhythm at 46 bpm. Superficial examination of the rhythm strip could lead to the erroneous diagnosis of SR with 2:1 A–V block; however, comparison of the first and last P–R intervals reveals that complete A–V dissociation is actually present. Note that throughout the rhythm strip, the alternate P-waves (B) remain too close to the preceding subjunctional beat to be expected to conduct, even if some A–V conduction were intrinsically possible. Since the heart rate is slow and the sinus rate is almost exactly double that of the subjunction, the relationship between the P-waves and QRSs changes quite slowly. It would therefore take many beats to shift the "B" P-waves far enough away from the Ts of the preceding beats to test whether some A–V conduction is possible. Remember that first-degree A–V block was present in the baseline ECG. Although apparently incapable of conduction, the "A" P-waves could conceivably have conducted with significant first-degree A–V block, had they not been preempted by the subjunctional QRSs. So, again, one must, in fact, wait for a P-wave to fall more toward the middle of electrical diastole in order to test the feasibility of A–V conduction.

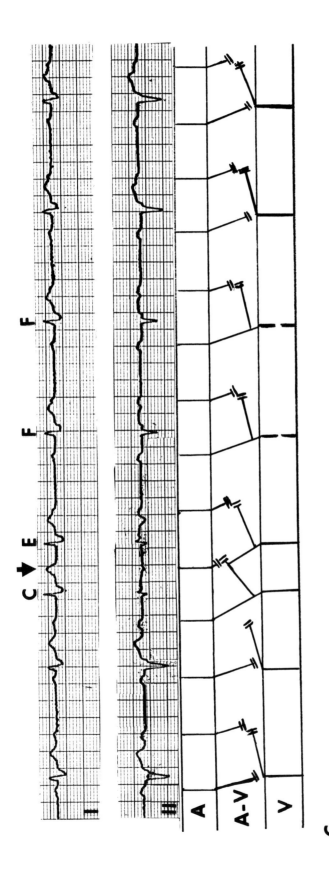

ECG II-35 (cont'd). C. A number of beats later, the P-wave has moved farther away from the previous subjunctional beat, and a capture (C) indeed occurs. A–V conduction is therefore intact. "Complete heart block" had never, in fact, existed. Prolonged A–V conduction and a critically timed escape rhythm resulted in prolonged A–V dissociation. The escape rhythm could easily have first appeared following an extrasystole or an A–V Wenckebach period. In this ECG, the escape pacemaker is located in the posterior fascicle of the left bundle branch, since the QRSs have the morphology of RBBB + left anterior hemiblock. What happens after the capture? The next P-wave (arrow) is followed by another supraventricular beat (E). This beat cannot be a capture, since its P–R interval is shorter than the P–R interval of C, despite the fact that its P-wave (arrow) sits atop a T-wave. We know from the many beats previously examined that such P-waves are incapable of conduction in this patient. E is therefore a *ventricular echo*. During the prolonged A–V conduction resulting in C, the antegrade impulse reaching the lower portion of the A–V node found another pathway recovered so as to conduct retrogradely. The retrograde impulse arrived in the highest reaches of the A–V node in time to collide with the antegrade impulse from the next sinus-P-wave (arrow). Before the collision, however, it found another pathway able to conduct antegradely, thus producing the ventricular echo (E). Because the retrograde impulse was unable to make an atrial echo (which would have appeared as a retrograde-P-wave), the ventricular echo is said to have resulted from an *abortive* or *concealed atrial echo*. The P-wave following E is unable to conduct either because of the intrinsic refractoriness of the A–V node, or because of an A–V node rendered refractory by concealed retrograde conduction in another attempt to make an atrial echo (the latter possibility is shown in the diagram). As the next P-wave is in the process of conduction to the ventricles, the subjunctional escape focus begins to fire. The result is a *fusion beat* (F). The P-wave following F finds the A–V node refractory, again, either because of intrinsic 2:1 block, or because of another concealed atrial echo. The next P-wave is timed so that a second fusion beat occurs. The next P-wave finds the A–V node refractory. The next P-wave's capture is completely preempted by the subjunctional escape beat. The next P-wave finds the A–V node refractory because of concealed retrograde penetration of the A–V node by the subjunctional beat. A–V dissociation then continues until a P-wave occurs sufficiently beyond the previous subjunctional beat for the refractoriness of the A–V node to have dissipated. Another capture can then occur.

A = Atria; A–V = A–V Node; V = Ventricles.

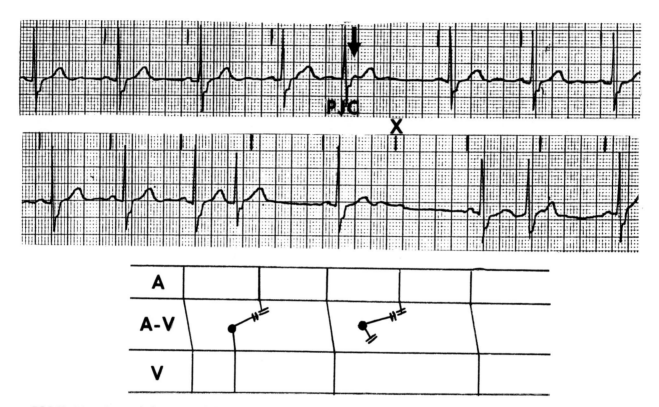

ECG II–36. *Concealed junctional discharge mimicking Mobitz II block ("pseudo-Mobitz II block").* These are two Holter monitor strips from a patient with frequent PJCs. Such a PJC is shown in the top strip. The sinus-P-wave (arrow) following the PJC is, of course, unable to conduct, since the junctional region is refractory. In the bottom strip, following the sinus beats, another PJC occurs. It is earlier than the PJC in the top strip, and has mild functional aberration. Again, the next sinus-P-wave cannot conduct. Following the next sinus beat, the P-wave (X) is suddenly nonconducted. Another, perhaps even earlier, junctional discharge occurred between the sinus beat and X. Because of the extreme "long-short" cycle ratio, this junctional impulse encountered functional trifascicular block, and did not produce a QRS. (Note that the long cycle of the "long-short" sequence is unusually long, since it consists of the pause following the previous PJC.) Despite the absence of a junctional QRS, X encountered a refractory junctional area and could not conduct.

A = Atria; A–V = A–V Node; V = Ventricles.

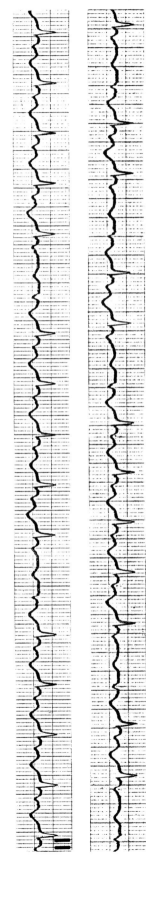

ECG II–37. *Mobitz II A–V block mimicked by an isoelectric PVC.* The basic rhythm is sinus tachycardia at 115 bpm. There are occasional sinus-P-waves which at first glance appear to be nonconducted; however, a T-wave follows each "nonconducted P-wave." Since ventricular repolarization requires antecedent depolarization, a QRS must be present. That the normal sinus-QRS was simply not inscribed because of some artifact is excluded by closer examination of these "isolated" T-waves. They are shallower and occur earlier than the sinus-T-waves. In addition, careful scrutiny of the "nonconducted P-waves" reveals their morphology to be slightly different from the morphology of the other P-waves; that is, they are slightly narrower and more pointy. The only phenomenon which could account for these findings is the superimposition of a virtually isoelectric QRS of a PVC on a sinus-P-wave. In contrast to the QRS, the T-wave of the PVC is not isoelectric in this lead.

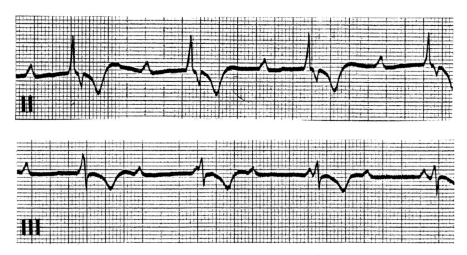

ECG II–38.   *Intermittent retrograde conduction in complete antegrade infra-nodal block.* Examination of Lead III reveals obvious complete A–V dissociation between the sinus (at 99 bpm) and a junctional escape rhythm (at 47 bpm). The cause of the A–V dissociation is advanced ("complete") heart block.

In Lead II, recorded immediately before Lead III, a retrograde-P-wave follows each QRS. Even more interesting, notice that the QRSs and the sinus-P-waves have a constant relation to each other; all the P–R intervals are equal. A–V dissociation is, in fact, not present in Lead II. There are two possible interpretations of this rhythm:

(1) The sinus-P-waves are conducted. The antegrade A–V block is intermittent. (Such "on-off" conduction is characteristic of infra-nodal block.) Marked P–R prolongation is present because of coexisting A–V nodal delay. Because of this delay, each QRS is followed by an atrial echo, which, in turn, resets the sinus.

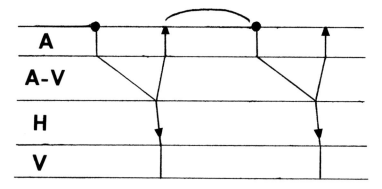

(2) There is still complete antegrade A–V block. None of the sinus-P-waves is conducted. There is a disparity between the ability to conduct in the antegrade and retrograde directions. Such antegrade-retrograde conduction disparity is common in the His-Purkinje system, and rare in the A–V node. The block is therefore located in the His-Purkinje system, and, considering the narrow QRS-complexes, in the bundle of His in particular. Each junctional QRS conducts retrogradely back to the atria, producing a retrograde-P-wave. Each retrograde-P-wave enters the sinus and resets it. In other words, the P–R intervals are all equal *because each sinus-P-wave is coupled to the previous QRS* via the retrograde P-wave.

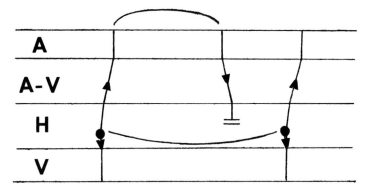

Since the R–R intervals in Lead II are identical to the junctional rate in Lead III, the second alternative is the correct interpretation. Such "reversed coupling" of a dominant pacemaker (in this case, the sinus) to a subsidiary pacemaker (in this case, the junction) is the explanation for periods of "fixed coupling" of a parasystole (see Section IV). Following failure of retrograde conduction, the sinus becomes uncoupled from the junction, resulting in complete A–V dissociation (Lead III).

A = Atria; A–V = A–V Node; H = Bundle of His; V = Ventricles.

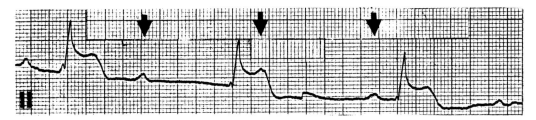

ECG II–39. *Advanced ("complete") A–V block in acute inferior wall MI.* There is coexistent sinus bradycardia (arrows) (43–45 bpm) and A–V block with a slow junctional escape rhythm (33 bpm). Such bradyarrhythmias reflect increased vagal tone, and are common during the early stages of an acute inferior wall MI.

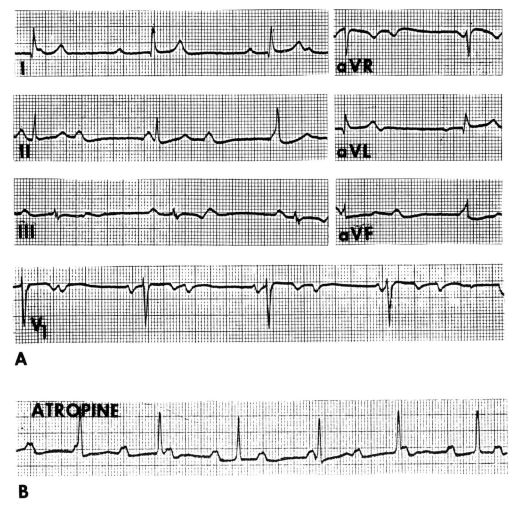

ECG II–40. *Congenital complete heart block.* A. The P-waves tend to be large; such atrial hypertrophy probably reflects life-long contraction occurring much of the time against closed A–V valves. B. Post-atropine, both the sinus and junctional rate increase, although complete heart block is still present. In congenital complete heart block, the site of the escape pacemaker is usually high in the junction, where it is subject to vagal influence. The junctional rate also increases with exercise.

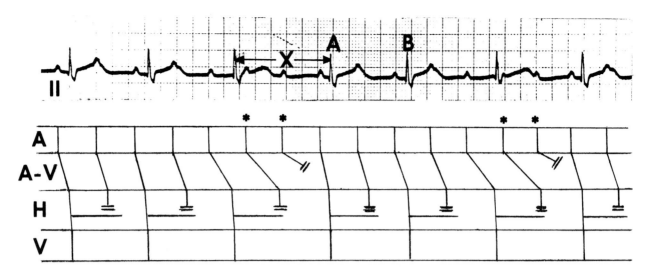

ECG II–41. *Bilevel A–V block.* The sinus rate is 130 bpm, and many nonconducted P-waves are obvious. The R–R intervals are irregular, with X being the longest. Although one cannot at this time say whether A is a junctional escape beat, all the other QRSs, which terminate shorter R–R intervals, are captures. On either side of X, one finds sequences in which the P–R intervals preceding the captures progressively increase, yet each is separated by a second, nonconducted P-wave. Assuming A is a capture (since it is preceded by a P–R interval feasible for capture, but which is shorter than the P–R interval preceding B), there are *two* nonconducted P-waves (*) during the X pause. The rhythm is therefore one of bilevel A–V block, in which the Wenckebach conduction occurs in the upper level, while 2:1 conduction occurs in the lower level. The upper level of block of course occurs in the A–V node. With an underlying atrial rate of 130 bpm, it is likely (though not certain) that the lower level of block is located in the bundle of His. (Halpern, M., et al.: Wenckebach periods of alternate beats. Circulation, *48*:41, 1973.)

A = Atria; A–V = A–V Node; H = Bundle of His (probably); V = Ventricles.

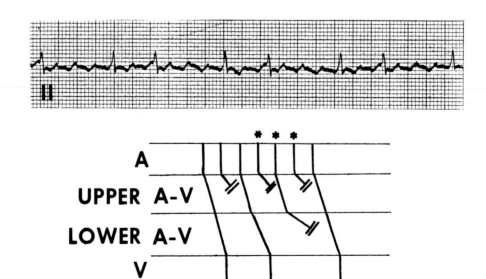

ECG II–42. *Bilevel A–V nodal block in atrial flutter.* The rhythm is atrial flutter with "2:1/4:1" A–V block. However, since the P–R (or flutter-R) interval preceding the long-cycle QRSs is different from the P–R interval preceding the short-cycle QRSs, the block is more complex, namely, bilevel. Since the long R–R cycles contain *three* nonconducted flutter-waves (*), the upper level of block is 2:1, while the lower is the Wenckebach, in this case 3:2. In such cases of atrial flutter, both levels of block are located within the A–V node.

A = Atria; A–V = A–V Node; V = Ventricles.

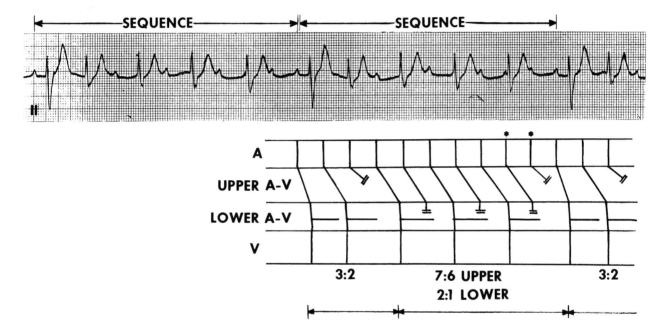

ECG II–43. *Complex A–V block: 3:2 alternating with bilevel A–V block.* The sinus rate is 144 bpm. After marking the location of all the P-waves, it is clear that many of them are nonconducted. The R–R intervals vary, yet two long, identical sequences (top brackets) are seen. A 12-lead ECG (not shown) revealed an acute inferior wall MI, with RBBB and intermittent left anterior hemiblock, the hemiblock tending to occur after long cycles ("bradycardia-dependent"). Three such bifascicular-block beats are seen in the rhythm strip. Each long sequence in the rhythm strip begins with a straightforward 3:2 A–V Wenckebach period. Following this, A–V conduction superficially appears to be 2:1. However, as in ECG II–41, the P–R intervals of the conducted P-waves progressively increase, finally resulting in *two* nonconducted P-waves (*). This portion of the sequence is therefore not 2:1, but *bilevel* A–V block. Since there are two consecutively nonconducted P-waves, the upper level of block is (7:6) Wenckebach, while the lower level is 2:1. Since typical 3:2 A–V Wenckebach periods are present, and the clinical setting is an acute inferior wall MI, both levels of block are almost certainly located in the A–V node.

A = Atria; A–V = A–V Node; V = Ventricles.

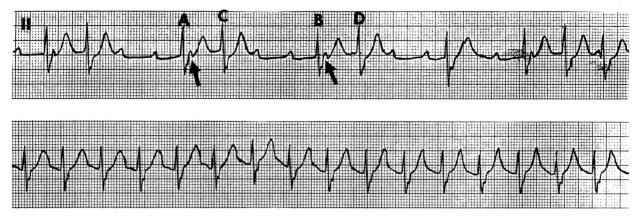

ECG II–44.   *Complex A–V block: A–V nodal reentry in the presence of advanced heart block.* The sinus rate is 120 bpm. There are many obvious nonconducted P-waves; advanced heart block is present. Since A and B, which terminate the longest (and equal) R–R intervals, are preceded by the same P–R interval, they are probably conducted beats. That this is definitely so is learned by examination of the capture beats (C and D) following A and B, respectively. The only P-waves (arrows) capable of producing these beats could not have captured if A and B had been junctional escape beats.* Therefore, A + C and B + D both constitute the beats of 3:2 A–V Wenckebach periods. The site of block is thus the A–V node. Suddenly, the heart rate increases to 110 bpm. During this nearly regular supraventricular tachycardia, complete A–V dissociation is present. By definition, since the tachycardia began suddenly, it is a paroxysmal tachycardia. The only rhythm it could be is a (slow) reentrant SVT. The reentry loop must be confined to the lower portion of the A–V node. The advanced, now "complete" A–V block must be confined to the upper portion of the A–V node. None of the P-waves can penetrate this zone of block to break the tachycardia, and the tachycardia cannot produce retrograde-P-waves. This patient was in the throes of an acute inferior wall MI, and this, in fact, is the same patient as in ECG II–43.

---

*If A and B were junctional escape beats they would have rendered the junctional region refractory; the subsequent P-waves, occurring so early, would have been blocked. Since A and B are, in fact, captures, the subsequent P-waves find the conducting system already recovered from traversal by the previous P-waves. Recall that if the sinus rate is fast and considerable first-degree A–V block is present, a P-wave can even occur slightly *before* a QRS and capture the *next* QRS (review ECG I–13).

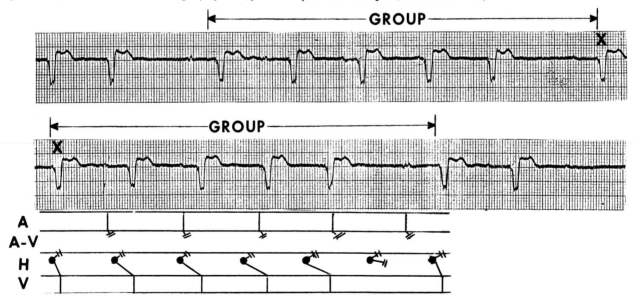

ECG II–45.   *Bilevel A–V block of advanced digitalis toxicity.* This rhythm strip was overlap-copied (X is the same beat). The sinus rate is 54 bpm. A–V dissociation is present. The R–R intervals are irregular, but careful inspection reveals two identical sequences (brackets). The QRSs are, in fact, *regularly irregular,* and constitute the *group beating* indicative of some type of Wenckebach phenomenon. The QRSs are related to each other, but not to the P-waves. Since some P-waves are in a position to capture, but fail to do so, A–V block is the cause of the A–V dissociation. There is a junctional rhythm with (6:5) Wenckebach block in His-Purkinje system, between the junction and the ventricles. Such block indicates advanced digitalis toxicity. (The serum digoxin level in this case was 8.0 ng/ml.) The junctional rate is calculated by dividing the interval containing the entire 6:5 Wenckebach period by 6, since a sixth junctional depolarization is present but nonconducted. The junctional rate thereby calculates to be 62 bpm.

A = Atria; A–V = A–V Node; H = Bundle of His; V = Ventricles.

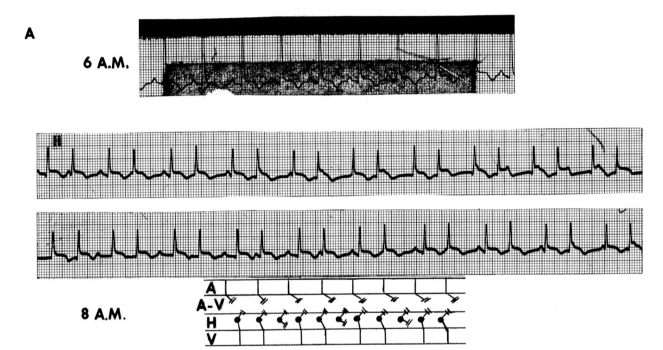

ECG II–46. *Bilevel A–V block with antegrade-retrograde conduction disparity in the A–V node.* This is a patient with an acute inferior wall MI. A. At 6 A.M., the rhythm was sinus at 95 bpm. At 8 A.M., the rhythm suddenly changed. A repetitive bigeminal supraventricular rhythm is present. The sinus rate has increased to 120 bpm. The P-waves are unrelated to the QRSs. Since none of the P-waves captures, A–V block is the cause of the A–V dissociation. There is complete block in the A–V node; there is a (markedly accelerated) junctional rhythm with 3:2 Wenckebach conduction in the His-Purkinje system. Dividing one bigeminal cycle by 3, one obtains a junctional rate of 180 bpm. The rapidity with which the junctional acceleration and advanced A–V block developed is much more characteristic of acute myocardial infarction than of digitalis toxicity. (This patient was not taking digitalis.)

A = Atria; A–V = A–V Node; H = Bundle of His; V = Ventricles.

B

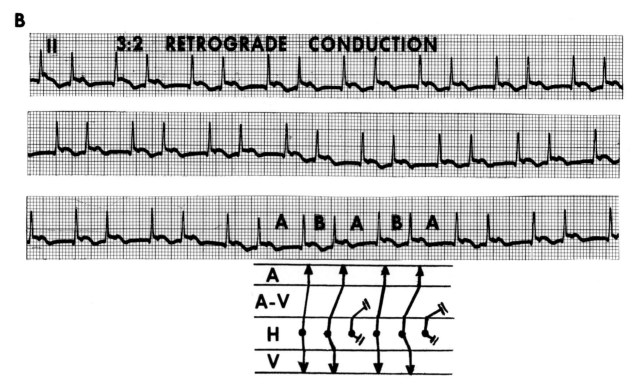

ECG II–46 (cont'd).   B. Several minutes later, periods of *3:2 retrograde conduction* through the A–V node occur. Note there are now retrograde-P-waves. All of the R–P intervals following the long (A) and short (B) cycle QRSs, respectively, are identical. The R–P interval within A is slightly longer than the R–P interval within B, indicating Wenckebach retrograde conduction through the A–V node or, possibly, the upper His bundle. Complete antegrade A–V nodal block is still present, since, upon the occasional interruption of the 3:2 retrograde conduction, thus producing the reemergence of the sinus, the previous rhythm shown in ECG II–46A would result. This disparity between antegrade (complete block) and retrograde (3:2) conduction is quite unusual in the A–V node.
    A = Atria; A–V = A–V Node; H = Bundle of His; V = Ventricles.

C

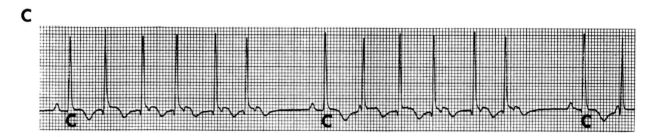

10 A.M.

ECG II–46 (cont'd).   C. By 10 A.M., the junctional rate, now irregular, has decreased to 126 bpm. H–V conduction has improved from 3:2 to 7:6. The sinus rate has decreased to 99 bpm. Antegrade A–V conduction is intact; the first beat in each sequence is a sinus capture (C). The sinus then becomes preempted by the junction, which subsequently conducts retrogradely to the atria, repeatedly entering and resetting the sinus. As in ECG II–46B, the fact that the antegradely nonconducted junctional beats simultaneously fail to retrogradely conduct (i.e., there is no isolated retrograde-P-wave during the pause) strongly suggests the junctional pacemaker is located high in the junction. The pacemaker's antegrade and retrograde output are thus both subject to a common, namely, vagal influence. The "H–V block" probably represents vagally mediated antegrade block (or exit block surrounding the pacemaker) low in the A–V node or high in the bundle of His.

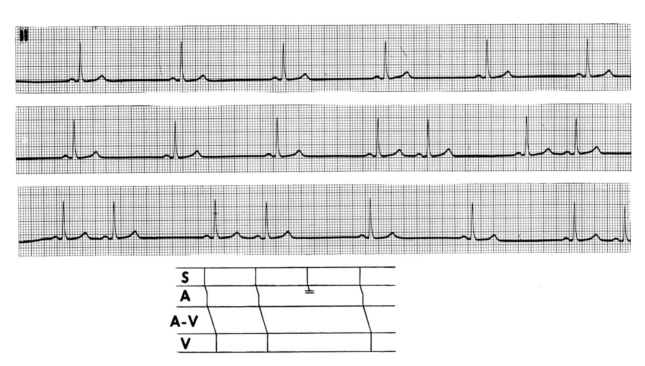

ECG II–47. *2:1 S–A block.* The P–P interval suddenly doubles.   S = Sinus Node; A = Atria; A–V = A–V Node; V = Ventricles.

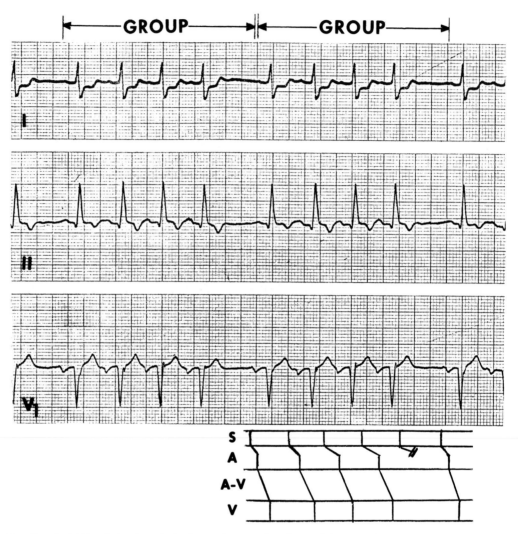

ECG II–48. *5:4 S–A Wenckebach periods.* Group beating (brackets) of the QRSs follows group beating of the P-waves; all P–R intervals are equal. The pause occurs when a P-wave is dropped. The sinus rate is 125 bpm.
S = Sinus Node; A = Atria; A–V = A–V Node; V = Ventricles.

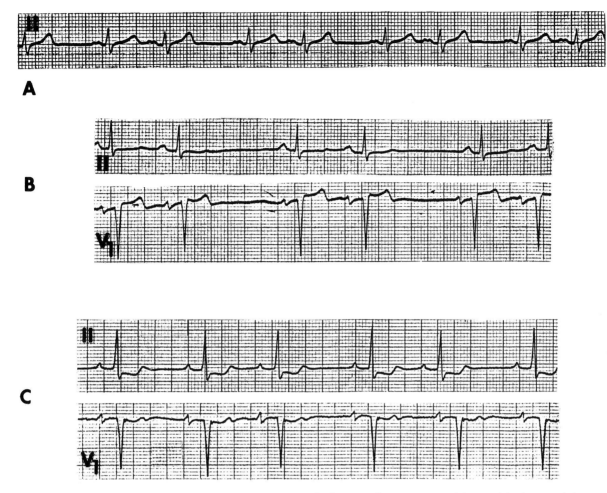

ECG II–49. *Three bigeminal rhythms.* A. 3:2 S–A block. The bigeminal pattern is repetitive, and the long and short cycle P-waves are identical. B. Peri-sinal PACs in bigeminy. The long and short cycle P-waves have slightly different morphologies. C. Pseudo-bigeminy in sinus arrhythmia. The bigeminal rhythm is not precisely repetitive, and, in Lead VI, finally breaks down.

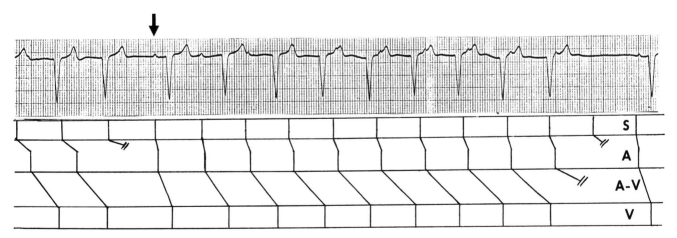

ECG II–50. *Coexisting S–A and A–V block.* First, mark off the P-waves. Notice that, beginning at the arrow, there is progressive P–R prolongation culminating in a dropped QRS. There is also group beating of the P-waves culminating in a dropped P-wave. There are therefore coexisting (11:10) S–A and (10:9) A–V Wenckebach periods. Since the S–A Wenckebach period is longer than the A–V Wenckebach period, the dropped QRS can occur. In contradistinction, when the A–V Wenckebach period exceeds the S–A Wenckebach period, the P-wave is dropped before the dropped QRS can occur. Such is the case of the sequence ending at the arrow.

S = Sinus Node; A = Atria; A–V = A–V Node; V = Ventricles.

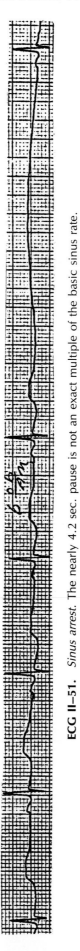

ECG II–51. *Sinus arrest.* The nearly 4.2 sec. pause is not an exact multiple of the basic sinus rate.

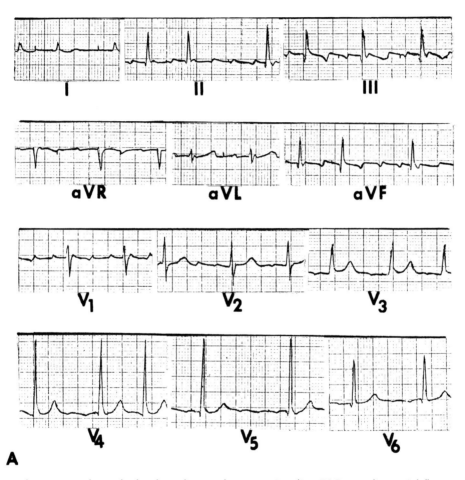

A

ECG II–52. *"Sick sinus" (tachycardia-bradycardia) syndrome.* A. Baseline ECG revealing atrial flutter with a moderate response. Note the small spikes of a nonfunctioning pacemaker.

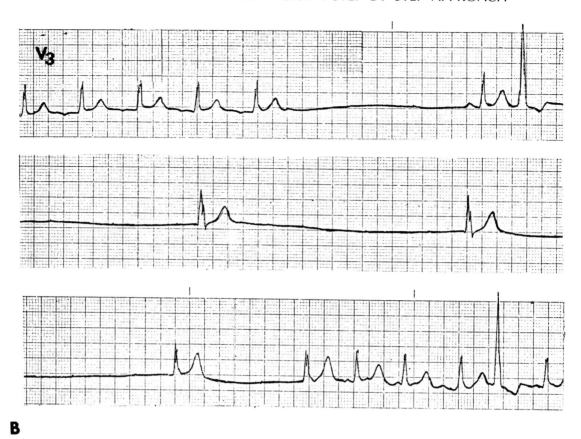

B

ECG II–52 (cont'd).   B. The reason for the pacemaker is now apparent. Following spontaneous termination of the atrial flutter, there is a long period of marked bradycardia during which an adequate escape rhythm fails to emerge. A single sinus beat escapes after 3.0 sec. Following a PVC, several junctional beats escape at approximately 16 bpm. Atrial flutter then resumes.

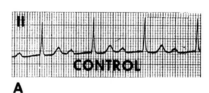

A

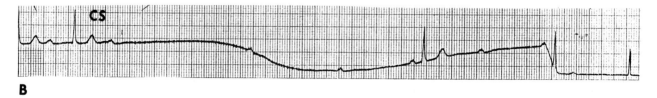

B

ECG II–53.   *Marked vagal surge resulting from a hypersensitive carotid sinus.* A. The baseline rhythm is sinus with first-degree A–V block. B. Following carotid massage (CS) there is a 5.6-sec. period of asystole produced by a combination of marked sinus slowing plus advanced A–V block. The site of block is the A–V node. (Reproduced with permission from Childers, R.: Classification of cardiac dysrhythmias. Med. Clin. North Am., *60:3,* 1976.)

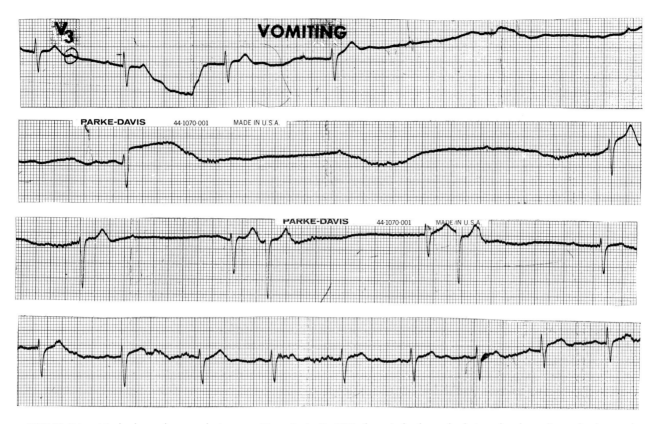

ECG II–54. *Marked vagal surge during vomiting.* As in II–53B, there is both marked sinus bradycardia and advanced A–V block.

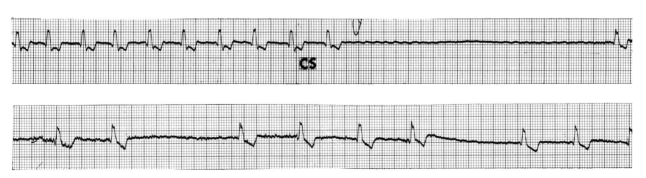

ECG II–55. *Carotid massage (CS) in a digitalized patient with atrial fibrillation.* Although the baseline ventricular response is moderately rapid, marked slowing occurs with carotid massage.

Ventricular Arrhythmias and Tachycardias with Wide QRS-Complexes

INTRODUCTION

You are triple-paged to the Emergency Room. You enter the Cardiac Area and see a half-dozen medical and nursing personnel rushing about in preparation for a cardiac emergency. Someone hands you an ECG. It shows a marked tachycardia with wide QRS-complexes . . .

This familiar situation represents one of the most anxiety-provoking and frequently difficult problems in clinical electrocardiography. Its solution requires prompt, but methodical, dispassionate analysis. Before embarking on a discussion of the differential diagnosis and methods of analysis, let us review the electrocardiographic characteristics of premature ventricular beats (PVC) and the various ventricular arrhythmias.

The PVC

PVCs arise ectopically in the Purkinje network in the ventricles, resulting from either enhanced automaticity (impulse formation) or localized reentry. Electrocardiographically, they produce wide (0.12 sec. or greater), bizarre QRS-complexes. When these beats are looked at in all twelve leads, they do *not* show classic bundle branch block (BBB) morphology (LBBB, RBBB, RBBB + anterior or posterior hemiblock). These classic patterns are reviewed in Figure III–1. Asynchronous activation of the ventricles *via* unusual activation sequences, along with the relatively slow spread of conduction through the myocardium, accounts for these features.

PVCs may have a single morphology (unifocal) or varying morphology (multifocal). Some authorities prefer the term *multiform* to multifocal, since recent ventricular mapping studies have demonstrated differing sequences of myocardial activation by a single ventricular focus; hence, some cases of "multifocal" PVCs really represent a single ventricular focus. Although not precisely conforming to classic bundle branch patterns, the morphology of the PVC may reveal the general location of the ventricular focus. Specifically, PVCs which generally resemble RBBB arise in the left ventricle; those resembling LBBB arise in either the right or left ventricle (this is explained by the fact that the ventricular impulse originates in the endocardium, and may first "break out" on the epicardial surface at a site distant from its origin).

The interval (coupling) between the PVC and the immediately preceding supraventricular beat may be unchanging ("constant" or "fixed") or variable. Unifocal PVCs with variable coupling may really represent a ventricular *parasystole,* which will be defined and discussed in Section IV. When a PVC occurs after every supraventricular (sinus or junctional) beat, *ventricular bigeminy* is said to be present (trigeminy if after every other beat). The coupling interval of a PVC may be short ("early" PVC) or relatively long ("late" PVC). A "PVC" that is considerably late may actually be an *accelerated ventricular escape* beat, and in the presence of underlying bradycardia, may be followed by subsequent beats of an *accelerated idioventricular rhythm* (AIVR; this will be discussed later).

As with atrial ectopy, a relatively slow heart rate

151

LEAD	RIGHT BUNDLE BRANCH BLOCK			LEFT BUNDLE BRANCH BLOCK
		+ LAHB	+ LPHB	
I	*	* or		
II, III, aVF	(Positive QRS-Complex)			(Positive or Negative QRS-Complex)
V₁		or		or
V₆		* or *		

*Small septal q-wave may be absent

Figure III–1. Classic bundle branch block patterns.

may predispose to ventricular ectopy ("Rule of Bigeminy"). In ischemic heart disease, rapid heart rates, by provoking ischemia, may also lead to the appearance of ventricular arrhythmias.

In sinus rhythm with a normal conducting system, a PVC may affect the subsequent sinus beat in one of four ways (see Figure III–2):

1. *Full compensatory pause:* The PVC conducts retrogradely into the conducting system. The next sinus-P-wave finds the conducting system fully refractory, and is therefore not conducted. It is the *following* sinus beat which conducts (normally). The R–R interval surrounding the PVC is therefore precisely equal to *two* sinus-cycle-lengths. In this, the usual case, the nonconducted P-wave occurs within the PVCs QRS-T complex, and may or may not be visible on the ECG.

2. *Partial interpolation:* Either (a) the PVC conducts retrogradely into the conducting system less extensively than above, and/or (b) the next sinus-P-wave occurs beyond the T-wave of the PVC, when the conducting system has partially recovered. This P-wave is therefore conducted, but with an *increased P–R interval*, so that the R–R in-

terval surrounding the PVC is equal to something *between* one and two sinus-cycle-lengths.

3. *Full interpolation:* The PVC barely penetrates the conducting system. The next sinus-P-wave encounters no conducting system delay, and thus conducts normally. The PVC therefore falls within precisely one sinus-cycle R–R interval.

4. *Retrograde atrial activation:* The PVC is able to conduct all the way back to the atria, producing a retrograde-P-wave. It, in turn, may or may not be able to antegradely conduct to produce a supra-ventricular QRS *(ventricular echo);* the longer the R–P interval between the PVC and retrograde-P-wave, the more likely the occurrence of the echo (see Section I). If a ventricular echo does occur, the R–R interval surrounding the PVC may be slightly shorter, the same (fortuitously) or slightly longer than one sinus-cycle, depending on the timing of the retrograde-P and subsequent P–R interval. With or without a ventricular echo, the sinus is reset by the retrograde-P.

Beats arising below the bifurcation of the His bundle, such as PVCs (in the Purkinje network) and subjunctional beats (in one of the bundle

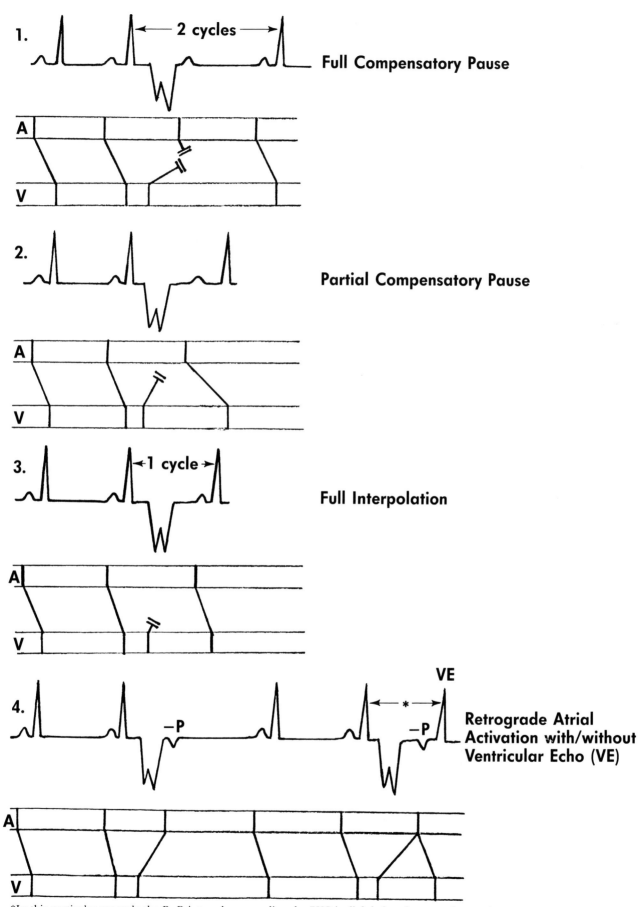

1. ← 2 cycles → **Full Compensatory Pause**

2. **Partial Compensatory Pause**

3. ← 1 cycle → **Full Interpolation**

4. VE
−P ←—*—→ −P **Retrograde Atrial Activation with/without Ventricular Echo (VE)**

*In this particular example the R–R interval surrounding the PVC is slightly less than one sinus-cycle.

Figure III–2. Effects of a PVC on the subsequent sinus beat.

153

branch fascicles) may, by virtue of their timing, be in *fusion* with a QRS of the dominant supraventricular rhythm. The initial vector (i.e., the direction and magnitude of the first 0.02 sec. of the QRS) of such beats may be either ventricular or supraventricular in origin. If the rhythm is sinus with PVCs, fusion beats preceded by a *shorter than normal* P–R interval have a different initial vector than the pure sinus captures, since the initial portion is from the PVC. Since a portion of all fusion beats is supraventricular in origin, the duration of such beats will be less than that of the corresponding PVCs. The earlier the PVC relative to the supraventricular beat, the lesser the degree of fusion. When a PVC arises from one of the ventricles near the site of BBB, a fusion of that PVC with the supraventricular beat produces a more or less normalized beat ("pseudonormalization"). In any fusion beat, the *T-wave* as well as the QRS is also in fusion, and is of a form intermediate between that of the supraventricular beat and PVC. To prove that a somewhat narrowed PVC is in fusion, one must see a P-wave in front of the PVC, measure the P–R interval of a pure sinus beat, and ascertain whether that P–R interval terminates during the duration of the PVC. If so, that portion of the beat beyond the termination of the P–R interval is supraventricular, and the beat is indeed a fusion.

PVCs may occur in salvoes: two in a row (a "pair" or "couplet") or three in a row (a "triplet"). Four or more PVCs in rapid succession are considered to be a short burst of ventricular tachycardia. The PVCs in these salvoes may be unifocal or multifocal.

Ventricular Tachycardia (VT)

This is a tachyarrhythmia characterized by long, often sustained salvoes of beats of ventricular origin (PVCs). It is generally a clinically dangerous rhythm, which may produce hypotension and low cardiac output, and may deteriorate into *ventricular fibrillation* (VF). Electrophysiologically, VT may be caused by enhanced ventricular automaticity, but, in most cases, it results from localized reentry within one region of the Purkinje network. Electrocardiographically, it is characterized by a tachyarrhythmia with wide, bizarre QRS-complexes which, in the same manner as an individual PVC, do not precisely conform to one of the classic BBB patterns. It may be regular or irregular, with a rate between 100 and 250 bpm. In a majority of cases, the rate is between 140 and 180 bpm. While most instances of VT are potentially dangerous, those which are more rapid (200 to 250 bpm), or which accelerate to such a rapid rate, are of particular

TABLE III–1. Electrocardiographic Features of Ventricular Tachycardia (VT).

1. Paroxysmal arrhythmia, rate 100–250 bpm (most cases between 140–180 bpm)
2. May be regular or irregular
3. QRS-complexes are 0.12 sec. wide (frequently more), and do not precisely conform to classic BBB pattern
4. Fusion beats may be present
5. May be interrupted by one or more sinus captures (early narrow-QRS preceded by a P-wave in a position to capture)
6. A–V dissociation during the arrhythmia may sometimes be discerned (P-waves may be both sinus and retrograde)
(7. Patient's hemodynamic status may or may not be compromised)

concern, since the repetitive falling of one beat's R-wave on the T-wave of the preceding beat ("R-on-T") may particularly enhance the possibility of VF. The electrocardiographic features of VT are summarized in Table III-1.

Ventricular tachycardia may begin with either an early or a late PVC. In sinus rhythm, when a PVC is late and/or the sinus rate is rapid, the PVC will be seen to preempt the completion of the normal P–R interval or the sinus-P-wave itself. When a tachycardia with wide QRS-complexes begins with such preemption, the diagnosis is VT.

During the course of VT, one or more fusion beats may occur. If a run of VT begins with a relatively late PVC, this first beat may be in fusion. Subsequent fusions may also be present. It is often possible to see a sinus-P-wave with a P–R interval appropriate for capture preceding the fusion beat. If one believes one has found many fusion beats throughout the course of ventricular tachycardia, one should "double check" by comparing the shortest interval between two adjacent "fusions" with the observed sinus rate before or after the VT. If the "fusion" rate greatly exceeds the known sinus rate, one is more likely dealing with respiratory or other variation of the QRS.

Occasionally a pure sinus capture will interrupt a run of VT. Such a beat is earlier than the expected ventricular beat, is preceded by a sinus-P-wave having a P–R interval appropriate for capture, and precisely resembles a normal sinus beat.

Although difficult or impossible to discern, the P-waves occurring during VT may be either sinus in origin, or may result from retrograde activation of the atria by the ventricular beat. Although pure cases of each occur (sinus-P-waves completely independent of the VT, VT with 1:1 retrograde atrial activation), in many cases of VT, the atrial activity is a combination of the two. Under these circumstances, intra-atrial electrode recordings reveal occasional *fusion P-waves*. Of clinical importance, however, is the identification of *A–V dissociation* during VT. When one is faced with a *paroxysmal* tachyarrhythmia (i.e., one that is observed to start and stop abruptly) of wide QRS-complexes, during the course of which discernible sinus-P-waves are seen to have no relation to the QRSs, the diagnosis is VT. Similarly, although occurring much less frequently, a *paroxysmal* tachyarrhythmia of wide QRS-complexes, during which Wenckebach or 2:1 retrograde activation of the atria occurs, is VT. Note that the word *paroxysmal* has been emphasized since either A–V dissociation or Wenckebach/2:1 V–A conduction may also occur during *nonparoxysmal tachyarrhythmias* with wide QRS-complexes, namely *accelerated junctional rhythm* (AJR) with BBB, or *accelerated subjunctional rhythm* (ASJR). Of course, one must observe the onset and termination of such tachyarrhythmias in order to ascertain their paroxysmal/nonparoxysmal nature. For example, in sinus rhythm, the paroxysmal rhythm (VT) begins as a premature beat preempting the sinus-QRS, and usually terminates abruptly. The nonparoxysmal rhythm (AJR, ASJR) appears only when the sinus becomes slowed or delayed below the junctional/subjunctional rate, and terminates either when the sinus again exceeds that rate, or when, during a period of A–V dissociation, the sinus-P-wave follows a junctional/subjunctional beat by an interval sufficient for it to be able to capture.

Ventricular tachycardia may be unifocal or multifocal ("polymorphic"); the form of the latter frequently involves a number of beats of one polarity in a given lead followed by beats of the opposite polarity. The two groups of beats may be separated from each other by several beats having an intermediate form ("torsade de pointes").

It must be emphasized that, while the occurrence of VT conjures up the vision of a desperately ill patient, one's hemodynamic status may in fact not be compromised during or by the rhythm. Experienced clinicians have all observed a patient sitting up, reading comfortably in bed in the CCU, while the monitor shows VT. One must never permit such a benign clinical picture from interfering with the proper electrocardiographic interpretation. A rough measure of the hemodynamic effect of a run of VT may be obtained by comparing the sinus rate before and after the run. If the rate has significantly increased, one can surmise a significantly lowered cardiac output during the arrhythmia.

Several further points must be made. The first is that it is possible for either PVCs or VT to appear as narrow QRS-complexes in a given lead. This may occur when either the initial or terminal portion of the QRS is isoelectric in that lead. When, particularly on a CCU single-channel monitor, an increase in the heart rate is accompanied by a slight change in QRS morphology or A–V dissociation, the possibility of VT must be considered. Other leads may reveal strikingly wider, more bizarre QRS-complexes, thus establishing the diagnosis. Secondly, again especially in the CCU setting, one must be careful about diagnosing gross ECG artifact as VT or VF. In these instances, despite gross deflections suggesting rapid QRS-T complexes, the patient's previous narrow QRS spikes continue undisturbed amidst the artifact. Finally, it must be mentioned that salvoes of *fusion-VT* may occur. If the supraventricular rate and the VT rate are similar, it is possible for long runs of VT to go undiagnosed. Here one looks for a slight change in QRS morphology (frequently observed as a decrease in the R- or S-wave) along with the intermediate T-waves.

VT usually responds to one or more of the various antiarrhythmic drugs. In the acute situation, intravenous lidocaine, procainamide, propranolol, and bretylium may be given (often in that order). When the VT is sustained, if either there is hemodynamic decompensation, or the various intravenous antiarrhythmic agents are not efficacious, DC shock is required to terminate the arrhythmia. DC shock is not indicated if the VT occurs in short, self-terminating paroxysms (i.e., is unsustained). Sustained VT also may often be terminated by short pacemaker-induced bursts of rapid VT. In addition, "overdrive" of the heart by pacing at faster than the spontaneous rate, may help prevent VT in drug-resistant patients, particularly if the underlying heart rate is slow.

Accelerated Idioventricular Rhythm (AIVR)

This rhythm is characterized by a series of two or more beats of ventricular origin, at a rate of 40 to 100 bpm. The morphology of the QRS-complexes resembles that of PVCs; that is, at least 0.12 sec. duration and not conforming to a classic BBB pattern. Normally, the latent pacemakers of the ventricular Purkinje network have escape rates of 35 bpm or less (see Section I). Under certain circumstances the escape rate of one of these pacemakers becomes enhanced to a rate between 40 and 100 bpm. Should the rate of the dominant supraventricular rhythm fall below the rate of this accelerated lower pacemaker, it will discharge, producing one or more escape beats. AIVR is a series of such beats, which may begin with an *early* or *late* PVC, or by an *accelerated ventricular escape* beat in cases of sinus slowing/delay or A–V block. It is usually observed in the setting of an acute myocardial infarction (MI), although it occasionally appears on ambulatory monitor recordings in patients having chronic heart disease. AIVR usually occurs in the presence of a relatively slow sinus rate (< 80 bpm). It may be regular or irregular, slightly accelerating ("warming up") or decelerating. It may terminate spontaneously, or when the sinus rate picks up and/or the P-wave is able to conduct and capture. Fusion beats often occur. During the rhythm there is frequently A–V dissociation, although retrograde capture of the atria by one or more beats may occur. In most cases, the duration of AIVR is between two and six beats, although longer runs may occur. Occasionally, true PVCs may occur in the middle of a run of AIVR; in most of these cases, the ventricular escape focus is reset one AIVR-cycle length from the PVC, although, in some instances, the escape rate of one or more post-PVC beats becomes additionally depressed. AIVR *per se* is a benign rhythm, although, occurring frequently during the first 12 hours of an acute MI, it may be temporally associated with the sinister ventricular arrhythmias, VT and VF. In rare instances, what is thought to be AIVR is in fact VT with 2:1 exit block; in these cases, a run of VT, with precisely the same QRS-morphology in all 12 leads and at a rate exactly twice that of the AIVR, occurs in temporal proximity to the AIVR. The beats of AIVR are usually unifocal in nature, since they represent a single escape focus; however, they may have the same morphology as the PVC which begins or interrupts the sequence, or which appears elsewhere as an isolated beat. To state the matter in another way, on a given rhythm strip, the same ventricular focus may appear as a PVC, VT, ventricular escape beat, or AIVR. In the setting of an acute MI, AIVR requires treatment if hemodynamic compromise results from the slow heart rate and/or loss of atrial systole; in such cases, the therapy is usually directed toward speeding up the sinus rate or ameliorating A–V conduction.

Ventricular Fibrillation (VF)

This rhythm, resulting from chaotic electrical discharges throughout the ventricles, is characterized electrocardiographically as a series of rapid, irregular, nonuniform undulations, without discernible P–QRS–T-complexes. Cardiac standstill occurs during VF, and, untreated, the initially coarse fibrillations become fine and finally disappear (flat line). In rare instances, a short run of VF may spontaneously convert back to a more stable rhythm. In the vast majority of cases, however, DC shock or, that failing, intravenous bretylium, is required to defibrillate the patient.

Ventricular Flutter

This is a relatively unusual rhythm, characterized by bizarre sinusoidal complexes at 300 to 400 bpm. As with VF, there is cardiac standstill during this rhythm. It tends to be short-lived, deteriorating into VF, usually within seconds.

Evaluation of Tachycardias Having Wide (≥ 0.12 sec.) QRS-Complexes

The differential diagnosis of tachyarrhythmias with wide QRS-complexes is summarized in Table III–2. Essentially, this encompasses VT, all supraventricular tachycardias (SVT), and ASJR. The electrocardiographic characteristics of VT, discussed earlier in this section and summarized in Table III–1, should be reviewed. The mechanisms and electrocardiographic features of the various SVTs discussed in Section I should also be reviewed. How and why may the QRS-complexes during these arrhythmias be widened? A SVT may have wide QRS-complexes because of:

1. *Pre-existing bundle branch block (BBB)*
   LBBB or RBBB with/without one of the hemiblocks had been chronically present. When the particular SVT occurred, the BBB merely continued. Examination of a previous ECG, if available, reveals one of the classic BBB patterns, the morphology of which is in all leads identical to that observed during the tachycardia.* Occasionally, the combination of BBB plus severe right ventricular hypertrophy (right axis deviation), or RBBB plus an old infarction pattern, renders the QRS-complexes bizarre. In such cases, SVT may

---

*The one exception is the rare case of complete LBBB with the QRS axis intermittently varying between normal and left axis deviation. In this case, both the previous and present ECGs reveal classic complete LBBB, but the QRS axis varies.

TABLE III–2. Differential Diagnosis of Tachycardias with Wide-QRS-Complexes.

1. Ventricular tachycardia (VT)
2. Supraventricular tachyarrhythmia* (SVT) with:
   a. Pre-existing bundle branch block
   b. Rate-related bundle branch block
   c. Sustained functional aberration
   d. Antegrade Kent bundle conduction
   e. Nonspecific QRS widening
      1. Hyperkalemia/acidosis
      2. Quinidine, procainamide, disopyramide
      3. Severe LVH or ischemia
3. Accelerated subjunctional rhythm (ASJR)

*These are reviewed in Section I

therefore mimic VT. Examination of previous ECG is necessary to make the differentiation.

2. *Rate-related BBB*

Above a certain heart rate, the diseased fascicle(s) can no longer conduct (or conducts extremely slowly), resulting in BBB. Presumably, the rate of the tachycardia exceeded that critical rate. Previous ECGs, if available, may or may not reveal BBB (i.e., the critical rate may not have been exceeded). However, if present, the BBB will be seen to have occurred at faster rates; in this case, as in (1), the QRS pattern should be identical to that presently observed.* Another possibility, combining the features of (1) and (2), is that an *incomplete* form of BBB** had previously existed, but now, at the fast rate of the tachyarrhythmia, conduction further worsened and the BBB had become complete. Previous ECGs, if available, reveal incomplete LBBB or RBBB; complete LBBB or RBBB, respectively, is now present. Or, RBBB (complete or incomplete) had been present; *complete* RBBB *plus a hemiblock* is now present. Whatever the case, the wide QRS-complexes conform to a classic BBB pattern.

3. *Sustained functional aberration (SFA)*

Although briefly mentioned in Section I, the

---

*The one exception is the rare case of complete LBBB with the QRS axis intermittently varying between normal and left axis deviation. In this case, both the previous and present ECGs reveal classic complete LBBB, but the QRS axis varies.

**Incomplete BBB resembles complete BBB, but the QRS duration is only 0.10 to 0.11 sec.

mechanisms of functional aberration (FA) and SFA will now be discussed. In most normal individuals, a relatively early supraventricular beat (PAC or PJC, or sinus beat following a junctional escape) encountering the His-Purkinje conducting system immediately after a relatively long R–R cycle-length may find one or more of the fascicles still refractory. This occurs because the refractory periods of the various components of the conducting system are determined by, and are directly related to, the previous cycle-length. Following relatively long cycle-lengths, the refractory period of one or more of the fascicles may exceed that of the A–V node, resulting in an early supraventricular beat's conduction to the ventricles, but with a BBB pattern. Such a beat would be said to have *functional aberration* of RBBB-type in most cases. Such RBBB may be complete or incomplete. Functional left anterior or posterior hemiblock (LAHB, LPHB) may occur alone or in combination with complete/incomplete RBBB. Complete/incomplete functional LBBB may also occur, but this probably happens less than 1% of the time; this low incidence of occurrence assumes great clinical significance, when one must decide between periods of SFA and VT during atrial fibrillation (soon to be discussed). The mechanism of FA is schematically shown in Figure III–3. As can be seen, when the appropriate "long-short" supraventricular R–R interval situation occurs, FA will result.

What of the mechanism of SFA? When a

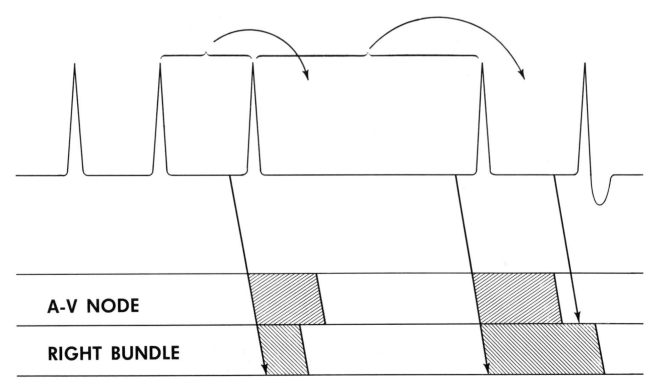

Figure III–3. Mechanism of functional aberration.

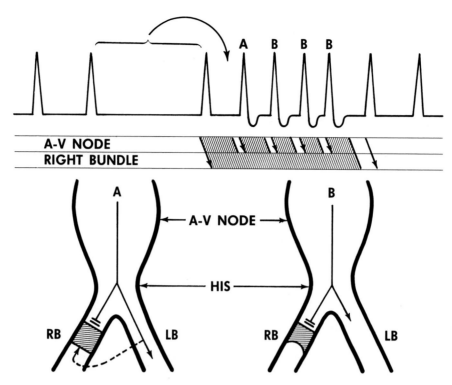

Figure III–4. Mechanism of sustained functional aberration.

"long-short" R–R cycle sequence producing FA is followed by one or more beats in rapid sequence (i.e., short R–R intervals), the aberration of the first beat may be sustained for one or more of the subsequent beats. The proposed mechanism is the concealed traversal of the interventricular septum, with resulting penetration and refractoriness of the bundle originally rendered functionally refractory. This is shown schematically in Figure III–4. As can be surmised, SFA, once established, will continue as long as (a) subsequent beats continue at a rapid rate, and (b) concealed transseptal conduction continues. Thus, each subsequent beat will continue to encounter a fascicle rendered refractory by the previous beat. If the rate slows down, allowing the conductivity of the affected fascicle to recover, or if one of the beats fails to traverse the septum, SFA will cease.

The first beat of SFA of complete RBBB- or LBBB-type may manifest incomplete BBB only. In the presence of atrial fibrillation (AF), this first aberrant, but narrower beat (0.10 to 0.11 sec.) may be mistaken for a fusion beat heralding a run of VT. In addition, in SFA of bifascicular type (RBBB plus a hemiblock), the functional block in one of the fascicles may be sustained for a greater number of beats than that in the other. In other words, FA or SFA of bifascicular type may convert to unifascicular SFA (RBBB alone or a hemiblock alone).

SFA may cease spontaneously, as previously discussed, or may be abolished by a critically

timed PVC arising on the same side of the heart as the blocked bundle. In the latter case, the PVC presumably enters the ipsilateral bundle, thus preempting its penetration by the transseptal impulse. As a result, the bundle will have recovered by the time the next beat occurs. Occasionally, SFA may be abolished by vagal maneuver. Obviously, a tachyarrhythmia which persists with narrow QRS-complexes after SFA has ceased is supraventricular in nature.*

A common, often very difficult problem in electrocardiography is the differentiation between runs of SFA and VT in the presence of AF. AF is usually a grossly irregularly irregular rhythm. However, during periods of rapid ventricular response (during which SFA may occur) differences between R–R intervals may not be easily discernible. Thus, by R–R cadence alone, runs of VT, which may be regular or irregular, frequently cannot be differentiated from a period of rapid ventricular response with SFA. Only if the run of aberrant QRSs is rapid and regular (or nearly so), amidst a *consistently grossly irregular slow*

---

*A unique circumstance occurs when a reentrant SVT with SFA *speeds up slightly* after the aberration has ceased. The mechanism is that the reentrant loop involves retrograde conduction through an accessory A–V connection (Kent bundle), which is located on the same side as the functionally blocked bundle. Antegrade conduction is *via* the A–V node and the contralateral bundle, thus creating an anatomically large reentry loop. When the blocked bundle resumes conduction (at the time of cessation of SFA), the size of reentry loop is greatly reduced, thus resulting in a speed-up of the heart rate.

or moderate ventricular response, is VT suggested.

The usually cited points for distinguishing between SFA and VT in the presence of AF are summarized in the left-hand column of Table III–3. Opposite each feature, in the right-hand column, are the reasons each rule may be fallible. Let us now consider each of these points.

"Long-short" R–R pattern: A "long-short" pattern is the prerequisite for SFA, but its presence does not necessarily mean SFA. A run of VT can also begin with a "long-short." In addition, in AF with a rapid response, the difference between the "long" and the "short" cycles of the "long-short" combination producing SFA, although discernible, may not be marked. So "eyeballing" the rhythm strip for a gross "long-short" pattern may be misleading. In summary, the usefulness of the "long-short" pattern is a *negative* one; namely, if it is absent, one is dealing with VT.

RBBB pattern of SFA: In 99% of cases of SFA, the QRS-pattern is that of a classic RBBB or RBBB plus a hemiblock. In the case of RBBB alone, the initial QRS-vector during the aberration should be identical to that of the narrow, conducted beats in all 12 ECG leads. In the presence of a hemiblock, however, the initial QRS forces may change in some of the leads. Specifically, if the conducted beats have a normal QRS-axis, small septal q-waves are frequently seen in most of the inferior and lateral leads of the frontal plane (I, II, III, aVL, aVF). If functional aberration of RBBB + LAHB occurs, the inferior leads develop initial r-waves (rS or rSs' pattern). If RBBB + LPHB occurs, the lateral leads develop initial r-waves (rS or rSs' pattern). In addition, in some cases of anterior or posterior hemiblock, the septal r-wave, seen in the right precordial leads, may be replaced by a small q (with the concomitant loss of the septal q-wave in Leads I and V_6); the presumed reason for these changes is the origination of the septal innervation from the blocked anterior or posterior fascicle. Finally, about 1% of the time, SFA is of LBBB type; in these cases, the initial QRS-vector may greatly differ from that of the conducted beats. If a run of beats having a LBBB pattern occurs, SFA is statistically unlikely, *but is not excluded.* Finally, it should be added that, in the absence of antiarrhythmic drugs or hyperkalemia, QRS durations exceeding 0.16 sec. are unusual in simple bundle branch block. If such extra-wide beats occur, despite conducted beats of normal width, ventricular origin can be presumed.

We can conclude that the key morphologic feature of SFA is that, whatever the type, *it always conforms to a classic BBB pattern* (review Figure III–1). In cases where the initial QRS-vectors of the aberrant and conducted beats are not the same, multiple leads (all 12 if possible, but certainly a lateral, inferior, right precordial, and left precordial lead) are required to accurately assess the nature of the aberration. Some examples of FA and PVC patterns, illustrating the above discussion, are given in Table III–4.

Fixed-coupling of first wide beat: This suggests VT; however, the first PVC of a run of VT often does not have fixed-coupling to the previous conducted beat. Furthermore, in AF with a rapid response, small differences between R–R intervals may not be discernible for several beats. If some of these beats are functionally aberrant, they may appear to be fixed-coupled.

Pause following the last wide beat: This favors VT; however, in AF with a rapid response, a pause may or may not occur after VT; in SFA, the aberration may have remitted *because* of a pause in the rate.

Presence of fusion beats: True fusion beats, of course, mean VT. However, in SFA, the aberration of the first beat of the run may be only par-

TABLE III–3. Sustained Functional Aberration (SFA) vs. Ventricular Tachycardia (VT) in Atrial Fibrillation (AF).

Differentiating Features	Fallacy
1. "Long-short" R–R pattern favors SFA	VT may also begin with an early PVC following a relatively long cycle-length
2. SFA usually has RBBB pattern (with initial QRS-vector identical to that of the narrow beats)	a. LBBB aberration occasionally occurs b. If the RBBB is accompanied by a hemiblock, the initial QRS-vector may not be the same as that of the narrow beats
3. Fixed-coupling of first wide beat favors VT	In AF with a rapid response, small differences between R–R intervals may not be discernible
4. Pause following the last wide beat favors VT	Pause may not occur if rate is rapid
5. Presence of fusion beats favors VT	The BBB of the first beat of a run of SFA may be incomplete, mimicking a fusion beat
6. Cycle-sequence comparison (see text) is reliable	Changing autonomic tone or concealed penetration of the affected bundle may invalidate the comparison

TABLE III–4.   Some Examples of Functional Aberration and PVCs by QRS Pattern.

Lead	Narrow (Conducted) Beats	Wide Beats	Comments
I *or* V₆			RBBB, same initial vector (LAHB may be present in "b")
			RBBB + LAHB / LPHB *or* PVC (must check other leads)
			PVC
			LBBB (*or* RBBB + LAHB if Lead I) *or* PVC (must check other leads)
V₁			RBBB, same initial vector
			PVC *or* RBBB + LPHB (must check other leads)
			PVC (most likely) *or* RBBB + hemiblock (must check other leads)
			PVC
			PVC *or* LBBB (must check other leads)
V₁			RBBB *or* PVC (must check other leads)
			PVC

tially developed (i.e., incomplete BBB), thus mimicking a fusion beat.

Cycle-sequence comparison: As previously discussed, a "long-short" R–R cycle is the prerequisite for FA. Suppose one finds a beat, X, believed to be functionally aberrant, and suppose the long and short cycles are of durations A and B, respectively. If, upon examination of the rest of the rhythm strip, one finds another long-short sequence, say C and D, respectively, then the beat, Y, terminating the short (D) cycle should also be functionally aberrant if: (a) Cycle C is longer than Cycle A (B = D), or (b) Cycle D is shorter than Cycle B (A = C), or (c) Both (a) and (b). If Y is not aberrant, when the long-short pattern is even more favorable for FA, then one must question whether the original beat, X, was not in fact a PVC, and not functionally aberrant (see Figure III–5). This method of analysis is called a *cycle-sequence comparison*, and is usually a reliable test. However, changing autonomic tone or the concealed penetration of the affected bundle during the long cycle by an atrial fibrillation impulse (thus making that bundle's long cycle less long than the visible R–R cycle) may occasionally invalidate such a comparison.

Although none of the methods for differentiating SFA from VT in AF is infallible, it can be stated that this differentiation is relatively straight-forward in most cases. The combination of (a) a long-short R–R sequence, (b) classic RBBB pattern with identical initial vector as the narrow beats, and (c) favorable cycle-sequence comparison is observed in the vast majority of cases. If either (b) or (c) is absent, one must examine multiple leads to determine whether the aberration precisely conforms to a known BBB pattern. If so, FA is highly likely; if not, one is dealing with VT.

Rarely, despite one's best effort, it is impossible to determine with surety whether one is dealing with runs of SFA or VT. In this case, *one treats the patient for VT,* keeping the following in mind: *Antiarrhythmic agents exacerbate SFA,* and usually suppress VT. Therefore, if, after administration of lidocaine or procainamide, the runs of aberrant beats become noticeably longer and/or more frequent, it can be concluded from this *therapeutic response* that one has been dealing with SFA.

4. *Antegrade Kent bundle conduction*

The mechanism for the Wolff-Parkinson-White (W-P-W) syndrome is reviewed schematically in

If beat X is functionally aberrant:

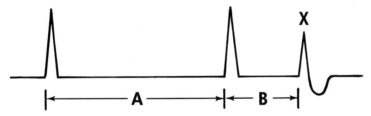

Beat Y should definitely be aberrant if:

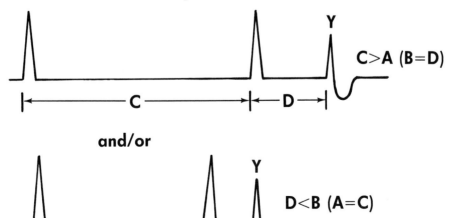

Figure III–5. Cycle sequence comparison.

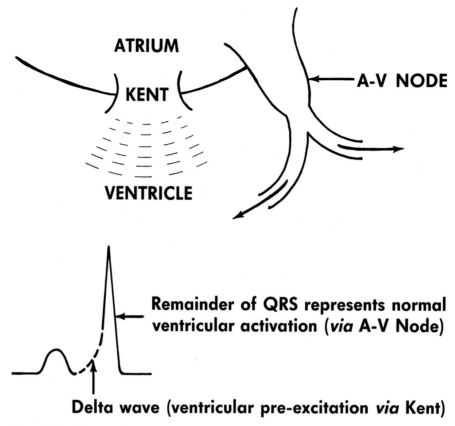

ATRIUM

KENT

A-V NODE

VENTRICLE

Remainder of QRS represents normal ventricular activation (*via* A-V Node)

Delta wave (ventricular pre-excitation *via* Kent)

Figure III–6. The Wolff-Parkinson-White syndrome.

Figure III–6. Essentially, antegrade conduction through an accessory atrioventricular connection, the bundle of Kent, results in pre-excitation of the ventricle. Since this pre-excitation results in asynchronous activation of the ventricles, a wide, bizarrely aberrant beat resembling a PVC begins to be inscribed. Usually, before completion of this beat, the remainder of the ventricles are activated *via* the normal conduction system. The resulting QRS is therefore actually a *fusion beat,* the first (or Kent) part of which is called a *delta wave.* The P–R interval is short (< 0.12 sec.), since the Kent conduction bypasses the A–V node and its delay. In patients with W-P-W, the following supraventricular tachyarrhythmias with wide QRS-complexes can occur (all involve antegrade Kent bundle conduction):

  a. *Sinus Tachycardia:* The heart rate is usually less than 150 bpm and sinus-P-waves are usually visible.
  b. *Reentrant SVT:* In the vast majority of cases the reentry loop involves antegrade conduction through the A–V node and retrograde conduction through the Kent bundle. Since the ventricles are activated by the normal conducting system, the QRS-complexes are narrow (review Section I). In rare instances, the loop involves antegrade Kent bundle conduction and retrograde A–V nodal con-

duction, resulting in wide, bizarre QRS-complexes. Retrograde-P-waves may or may not be discernible. The tachycardia is regular, and the heart rate is usually 150 to 250 bpm. Previous ECGs, if available, reveal delta waves. In every lead, the delta waves should match the initial portion of the present aberrant QRS-complexes. Vagal maneuvers are almost always successful in breaking the rhythm, again revealing delta waves when sinus rhythm resumes.

  c. *Atrial Fibrillation and Atrial Flutter:* Without the usual A–V nodal delay, the ventricular response can be up to 300 to 350 bpm. In fact, the point should be made: Whenever one has a wide-complex tachyarrhythmia in which the heart rate ever reaches or exceeds 300 bpm, atrial fibrillation or flutter with antegrade Kent bundle conduction becomes, by far, the most likely diagnosis. Given a less conductive Kent bundle, the heart rate, of course, will be less. Occasional narrow beats or intermediate (fusion) beats (with delta waves) may occur. At rates below 300 bpm, the differentiation between AF with antegrade Kent conduction and VT (which may also have some narrow beats [pure captures and fusions]) lies in the gross irregularity of the former. In AF, one expects at least some periods of gross irregularity, with the length of some R–R intervals two to three times that of others. This degree of irregularity is not seen in VT. Drugs like lidocaine, procainamide, and aprindine may further block the Kent bundle, resulting in slower ventricular response.

5. *Non-specific QRS Widening*

As indicated in Table III–2, the principal causes of non-specific QRS widening are (a) hyperkalemia/acidosis, (b) antiarrhythmic agents (quinidine, procainamide, disopyramide), and (c) severe left ventricular hypertrophy/ischemia. In each of these cases, the QRS-complexes are wide ($\geq$ 0.12 sec., frequently > 0.16 sec.), bizarre, and do not conform to a typical BBB pattern. Any SVT, particularly marked sinus tachycardia or atrial fibrillation/flutter with a rapid response, may mimic VT. In each of these cases, the underlying atrial rhythm may sometimes be discerned. The patient may give a history of antiarrhythmic drugs, or may have the physical/laboratory findings of metabolic acidosis. Previous ECGs may reveal progressive QRS widening along the morphologic lines of the presently observed complexes. In the case of clinical acidosis/hyperkalemia, the QRS-complexes will narrow in front of one's eyes following intravenous administration of calcium or sodium bicarbonate, and restoration of the serum pH.

It must be mentioned that patients likely to have non-specific QRS widening from the above causes are also highly susceptible to VT (e.g., from unsuccessful treatment by, or idiosyncratic or toxic reaction to antiarrhythmic drugs; from

acidosis; etc.). In addition, severe hyperkalemia or ischemia may occasionally produce *classic BBB*. The QRS duration in these cases is usually particularly wide (> 0.16 sec.), reflecting the underlying problem.

Accelerated Subjunctional Rhythm (ASJR)

This rhythm represents a nonparoxysmal acceleration of a latent subsidiary pacemaker of the heart. It differs from AJR, discussed in Section I, only in that the pacemaker focus is located in the proximal portion of one of the bundle fascicles, rather than in the His bundle or N–H region of the A–V node. The causes of ASJR are identical to those of AJR (review Table I–7). In this rhythm, the QRS-complexes conform to a classic BBB pattern. Since the rhythm originates below the bifurcation of the His bundle, fusion beats may occur. During the rhythm there may be A–V dissociation, or various varieties of V–A conduction, including 1:1, Wenckebach, and, rarely, 2:1 types. It is a *nonparoxysmal tachycardia,* appearing only when the sinus is slowed or delayed below the subjunctional pacemaker rate, or when A–V block is present. It disappears only when the sinus picks up and is in a position to capture (i.e., does not fall within or immediately after the QRS-T of the previous subjunctional beat), or when A–V conduction improves, or when the rate of the subjunctional pacemaker decelerates. (Unlike a paroxysmal arrhythmia, which suddenly stops, this deceleration is a gradual process, taking many hours or days.)

LEAD V$_2$

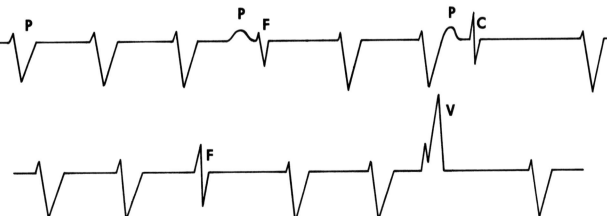

Upper Panel: VT. A pure supraventricular capture (C), as well as a fusion beat (F), is present. Both are preceded by P-waves with a P–R interval appropriate for capture. These P-waves are often discernible.

Lower Panel: SVT with BBB. A pure PVC (V) with opposite BBB pattern, as well as a fusion beat (F), is present. Neither is preceded by a discernible P-wave.

Figure III–7. Regular wide-QRS tachycardias with occasional narrow beats.

TABLE III–5. Diagnostic Approach to Tachycardias with Wide-QRS-Complexes.

1. Previous ECG
   a. Presence of BBB or delta waves → SVT with BBB or antegrade Kent conduction
   b. Previous PVCs, short runs of VT having same morphology as present wide-QRS → VT
   c. Progressive widening of QRS along same morphologic lines as present wide-QRS → SVT with nonspecific QRS widening
   d. Slightly accelerated subjunction or foreshortened escape time → ASJR
2. Present ECG
   a. True fusion beats → VT *or* ASJR *or* AF with W-P-W
   b. QRS aberration does not conform to classic BBB patterns → VT *or* SVT with antegrade Kent conduction or nonspecific QRS widening
   c. Ventricular rate 300–350 bpm → atrial flutter or fibrillation with antegrade Kent conduction
   d. A–V dissociation or variable (Wenckebach or 2:1) V–A conduction →
      i. VT if *paroxysmal* with *atypical* QRS widening
      ii. ASJR if *nonparoxysmal* with *classic BBB* pattern
   e. If rhythm briefly breaks, observe:
      i. QRS morphology of conducted beats (for BBB, delta waves)
      ii. Presence of PVCs or single PACs with functional aberration (similar QRS morphology)
      iii. How does tachycardia restart? (e.g., does it begin by an obvious PAC or PVC?)
   f. Regular wide-QRS tachycardia with occasional fusion beats:
      i. Pure supraventricular captures present → VT with fusion beats
      ii. Pure PVCs with opposite BBB morphology → SVT with BBB
3. Therapeutic interventions
   a. Vagal maneuvers (carotid massage, Tensilon, etc.): These may slow the ventricular response, allowing underlying atrial activity to be seen. They may also abolish some SVTs, particularly reentrant SVT. Finally, they may occasionally abolish SFA while not terminating the tachycardia
   b. Antiarrhythmic drugs (lidocaine, procainamide): These will abolish or improve most cases of VT, but will exacerbate SFA

Junctional or subjunctional rhythm is considered accelerated when the rate exceeds 60 bpm; it rarely exceeds 160 bpm. Obviously, difficulty in differentiation from other tachyarrhythmias tends to occur only when the rate is markedly accelerated (120 to 160 bpm).

Regular Wide-QRS Tachycardias with Occasional Fusion Beats

This rhythm may be (a) VT, occasionally narrowed by fusion with supraventricular captures,* or (b) SVT with BBB, occasionally normalized by fusion with ipsilateral PVCs (see Figure III–7). In the case of (a), pure captures are often present. They are identified as narrow, normal-looking QRS-complexes occurring too early to be fusions. Both the pure captures and fusions (which are of

intermediate morphology and duration) often follow discernible P-waves (by a P–R interval appropriate for capture). In the case of (b), pure PVCs are often observed, and are identified as early wide-QRS-complexes having a BBB morphology opposite to that of the dominant rhythm. Neither the fusions nor pure PVCs are preceded by discernible P-waves. In addition, it must be again emphasized that SVT with BBB conforms to a classic BBB pattern; VT does not.

Summary

Now that the various arrhythmias producing tachycardias with wide-QRS-complexes have been discussed, let us summarize in Table III–5 our diagnostic approach. The key elements are careful and methodical analysis, maximal use of data (multiple ECG leads, previous ECGs, etc.), and, not infrequently, observation of the effects of therapy (vagal maneuvers, antiarrhythmic agents, etc.). Adherence to these principles results in the correct diagnosis in almost every instance.

---

*While, in most instances, a supraventricular capture represents an antegrade *sinus capture*, it may occasionally be a *ventricular echo*, resulting from prolonged V–A conduction during the VT. In the latter case, the capture is preceded by a *retrograde-P-wave*.

SECTION III
Electrocardiograms

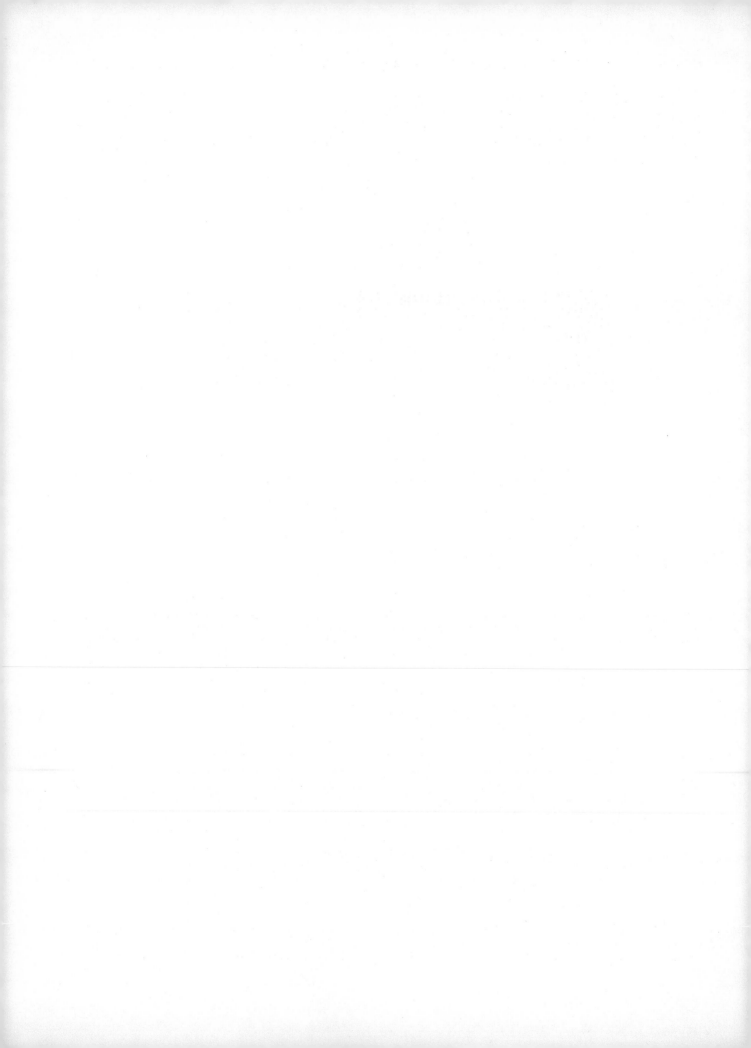

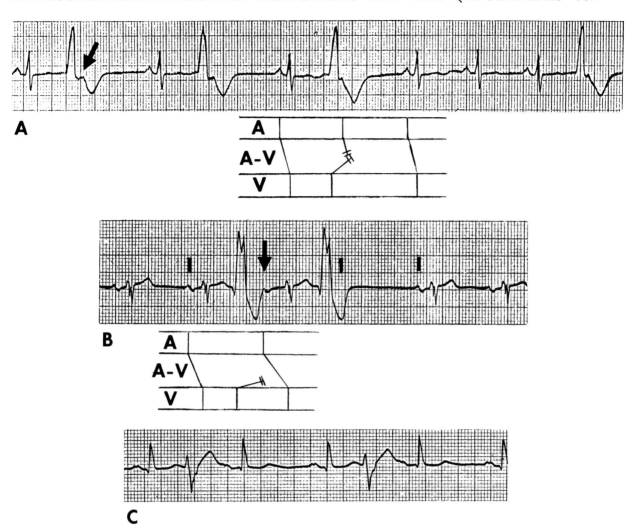

ECG III–1. *Unifocal, fixed-coupled PVCs:* A. Full compensatory pause. The P-wave (arrow) following each PVC does not conduct. There is concealed retrograde penetration of the A–V node by the PVC, rendering it refractory to the subsequent P-wave. B. Partial interpolation. The P-wave (arrow) following the first PVC conducts, but with first-degree A–V block. This P-wave finds the conducting system partially refractory, because of concealed retrograde conduction by the PVC. In this case, the retrograde penetration of the node is less deep than in III–1A. The P-wave following the second PVC is buried in the PVCs T-wave, and does not conduct. C. Partial interpolation. The P-wave following each PVC conducts with mild first-degree A–V block.

A = Atria; A–V = A–V Node; V = Ventricles.

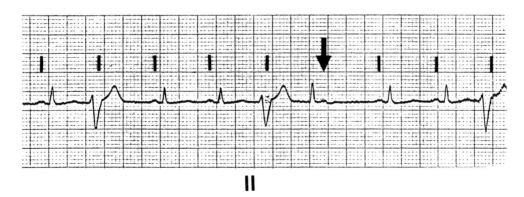

ECG III–2. *Partially interpolated PVC producing a dropped beat.* Unifocal fixed-coupled PVCs are present. The first PVC is followed by a full compensatory pause. The second PVC is partially interpolated; the P-wave buried within the PVC conducts with marked first-degree A–V block. The next P-wave (arrow) follows in close order and cannot conduct.

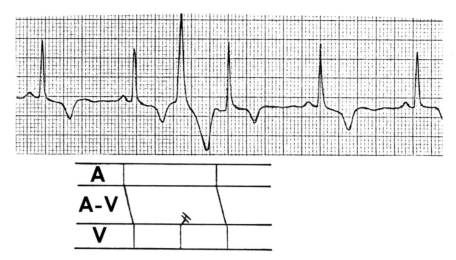

ECG III–3.   *Fully interpolated PVC.* The R–R interval surrounding the PVC is equal to the others. Presumably, there was only minimal retrograde penetration of the conducting system by the PVC.
A = Atria; A–V = A–V Node; V = Ventricles.

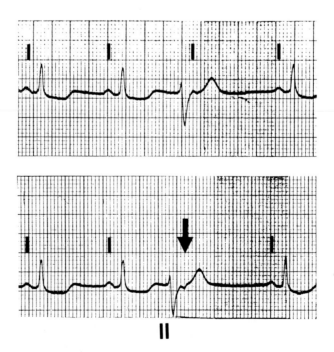

ECG III–4.   *Unifocal PVCs with and without complete V–A conduction.* The PVC in the top strip is followed by a full compensatory pause. This PVC retrogradely penetrated the conducting system, rendering it refractory to the next sinus-P-wave. In the bottom strip, the PVC succeeded in retrogradely conducting all the way back to the atria, producing a retrograde-P-wave (arrow). The sinus is then reset.

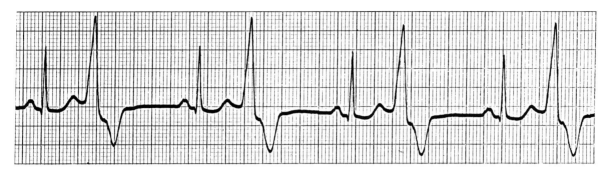

ECG III–5. *Unifocal fixed-coupled PVCs in bigeminy.* In this particular case, the true sinus rate is not known. The rate could be 37 bpm or 74 bpm. If the latter case, the second, nonconducted P-waves are completely buried within the ST–T complex. (Stein, E. *The Electrocardiogram: A Self-Study Course in Clinical Electrocardiography.* Courtesy of W. B. Saunders Co., 1976.)

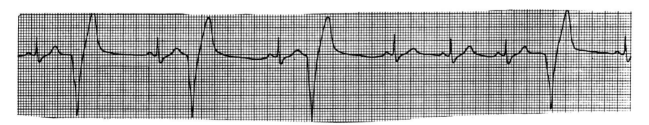

ECG III–6. *Unifocal non-fixed-coupled PVCs.* Such PVCs may represent a ventricular *parasystole,* that is, a latent ventricular pacemaker which has acquired entrance block so that it is no longer suppressed by the faster sinus (see Section IV).

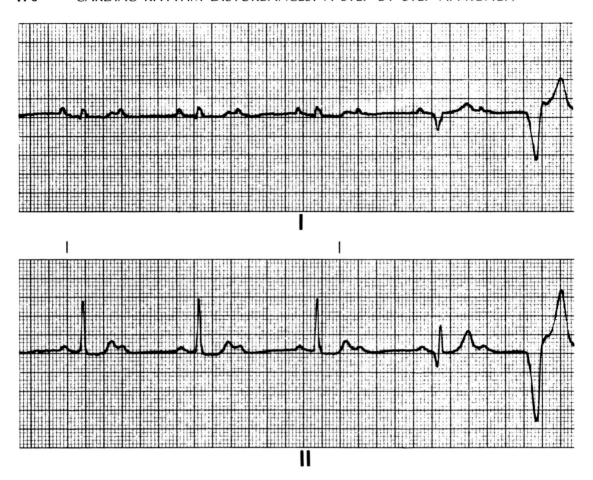

ECG III–7. *PVC in fusion.* The first of the two PVCs is in fusion. The underlying rhythm is sinus with 2:1 A–V block. Simultaneous Leads I and II.

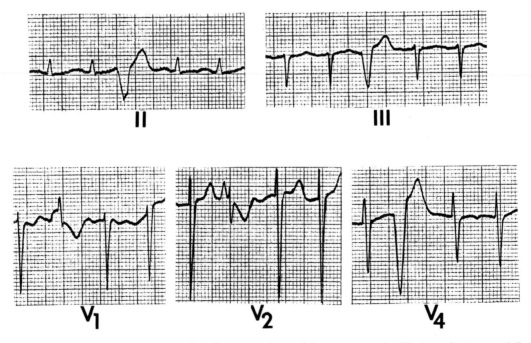

ECG III–8. *PVC mimicking a PAC.* In Lead V_2 the morphology of the PVC gives the illusion of a P-wave followed by a narrow, though aberrant QRS.

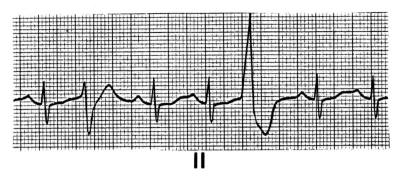

ECG III–9. *Multiforme PVCs.* The two PVCs have different morphologies.

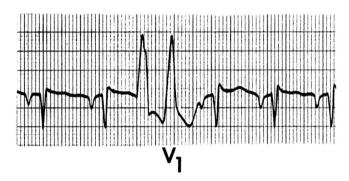

ECG III–10. *PVC couplet (pair).*

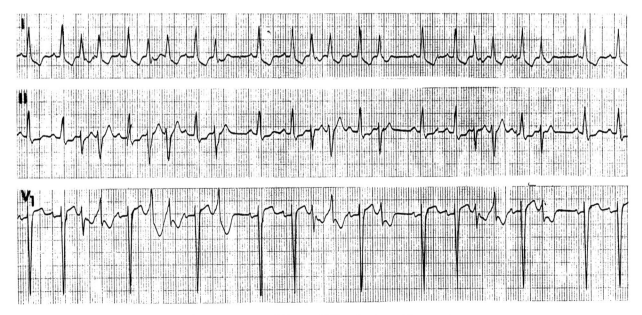

ECG III–11. *Multiforme PVCs, singly and in couplets.*

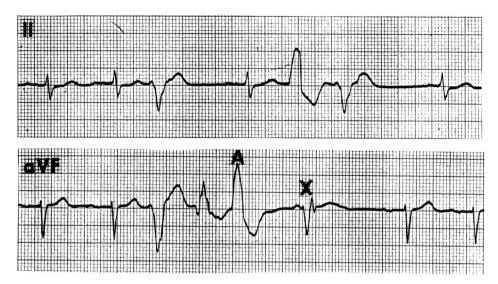

ECG III–12. *Multiforme PVCs, including one couplet and triplet.* The triplet is followed by a late PVC (X). X should not be included with the triplet, since the interval between A and X is long (i.e., greater than 600 msec.).

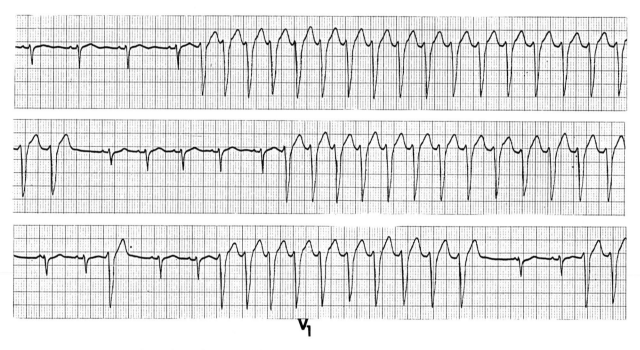

ECG III–13. *Ventricular tachycardia (VT).* In this case, the VT is unifocal at approximately 150 bpm. It slightly decelerates, once begun. Note the single PVC having the same morphology as the VT.

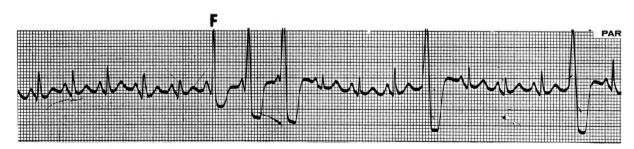

ECG III–14. *Unifocal PVCs, including a triplet.* The triplet begins with a fusion beat (F). During the triplet, A–V dissociation is evident.

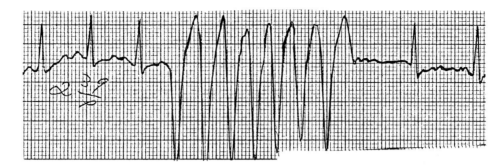

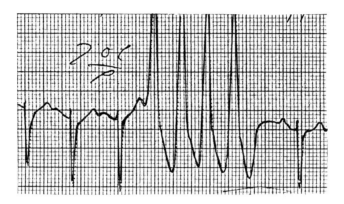

A

ECG III–15. *Rapid VT.* A. The rate is approximately 220 bpm.

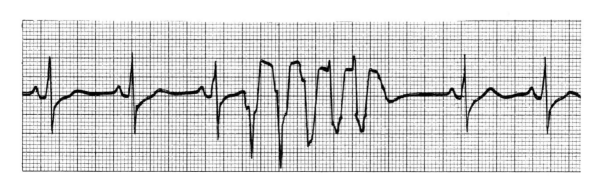

B

ECG III–15 (cont'd). B. The rate accelerates to approximately 220 bpm.

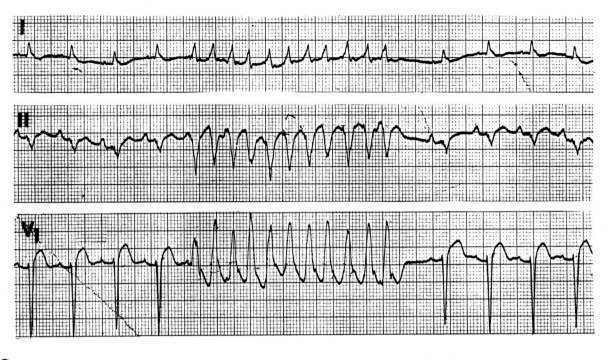

C

ECG III–15 (cont'd).   C. The first beat preempts the normally occurring P-wave. Note how the PVCs resemble the supraventricular beats in Lead I.

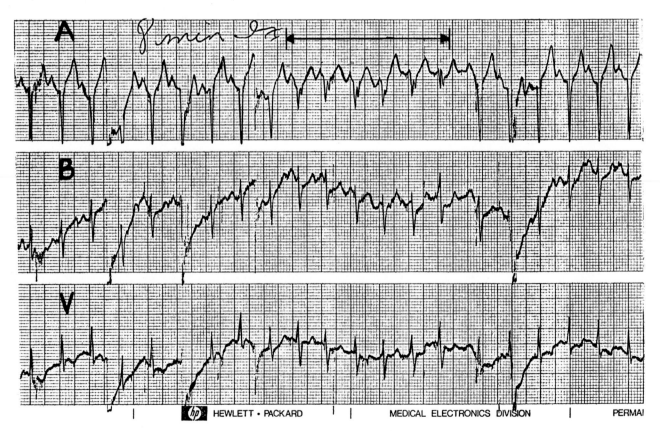

ECG III–16.   *VT during exercise.* In Lead A the VT is readily identified (bracket) by the different QRS morphology and the presence of A–V dissociation. This obviously important rhythm would probably have been missed if only Leads B and V were perused.

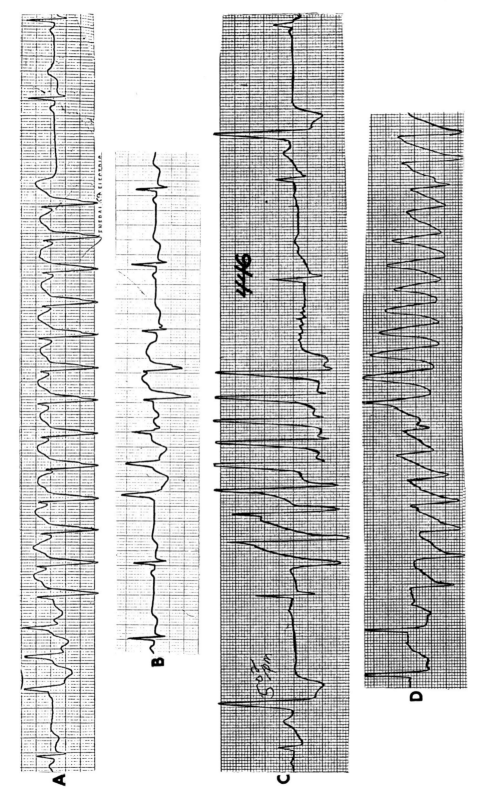

ECG III–17. A–D. *Multiforme VT.* Examples B–D, in which the upright and negative QRSs are separated by transitional complexes, are called "torsade de pointes." (Prolonged Q–T intervals are often found in the supraventricular beats.) The usual causes are (1) congenital Q–T prolongation syndrome and (2) Type I antiarrhythmic drugs (toxicity or idiosyncratic reaction). Pacing the heart at a faster than the intrinsic sinus rate frequently suppresses the ventricular tachycardia (overdrive suppression).

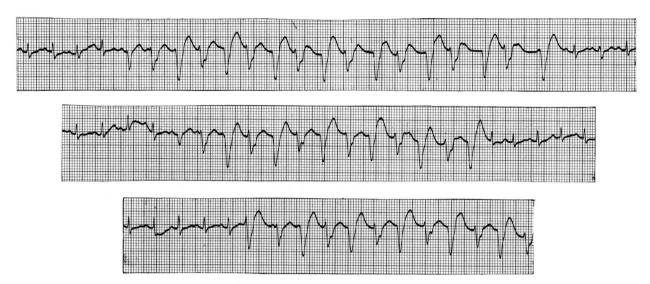

ECG III–18. *Alternating QRSs in VT.* There is alternation of both QRS morphology and interectopic interval.

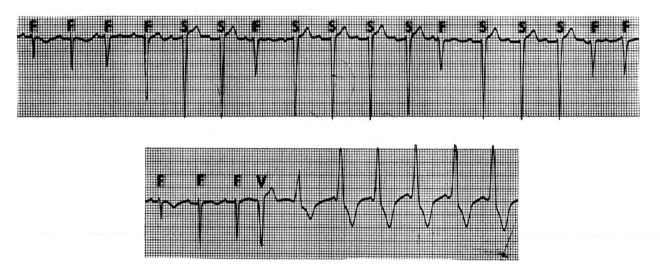

ECG III–19. *Fusion-VT.* The pure sinus beats are labeled S. These consist of negative QRS-complexes and upright T-waves. There are salvoes of slow VT, consisting of upright QRS-complexes and negative T-waves. (One PVC [V] from another focus is present.) There are many fusion beats (F), consisting of intermediate QRS-complexes and T-waves. A run of such fusion beats, of course, represents a run of VT in fusion with the supraventricular beats, which occur at approximately the same rate.

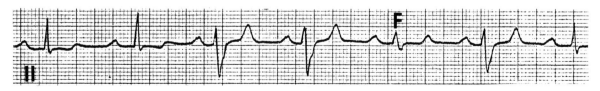

ECG III–20. *Accelerated idioventricular rhythm (AIVR).* The 4-beat run begins with a late PVC and continues at 60 bpm. The third beat of the run is a fusion beat (F).

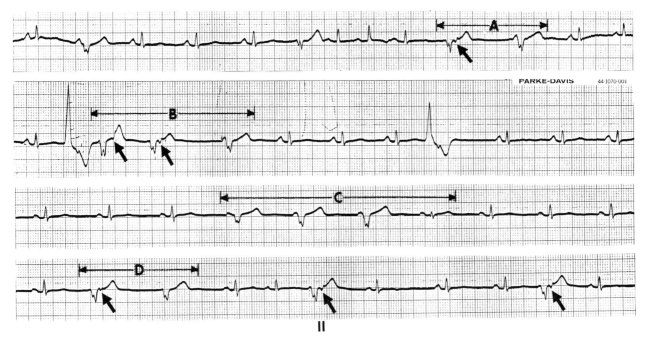

ECG III–21. *AIVR beginning with both early and late PVCs.* The basic rhythm is sinus with PACs. A number of PVCs are present. Two to four-beat runs of AIVR (brackets) are present. A and D begin with relatively early PVCs; B begins with the second PVC of a multiforme couplet. C begins with a late PVC; in fact, the first and fourth beat of the sequence are fusions. A number of beats conduct retrogradely to the atria (arrows).

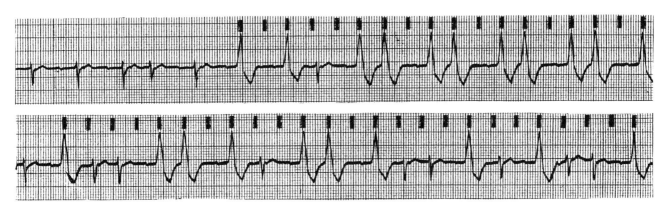

ECG III–22. *VT with exit block.* The longer interectopic intervals are all multiples of the shortest one. The underlying rhythm is AF.

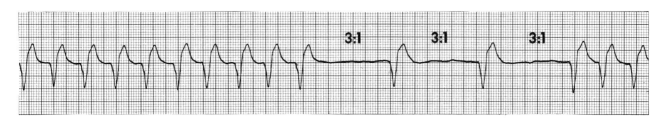

ECG III–23. *VT with exit block.* The underlying rhythm is flat line. This patient took a fatal overdose of digoxin.

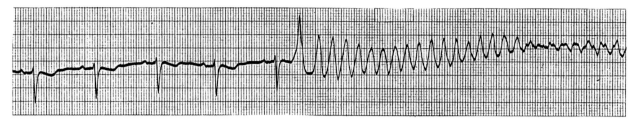

ECG III–24. *Ventricular fibrillation (VF).* The VF is triggered by an "R-on-T" PVC.

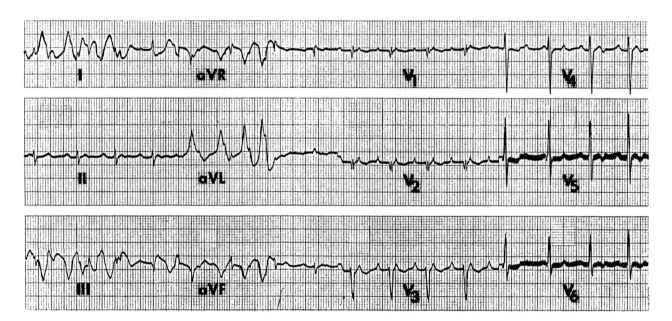

ECG III–25. *Artifactual VT.* Lead II is unaffected by the artifact.

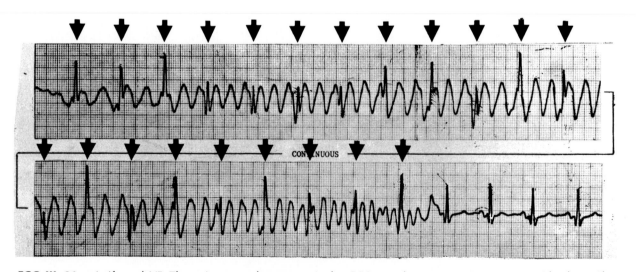

ECG III–26. *Artifactual VF.* The uninterrupted supraventricular QRS-complexes (arrows) are seen amidst the artifact. (From DeSanctis, R., Block, P., and Hutter, A. Tachyarrhythmias in myocardial infarction. Circulation, *45*:681, 1972. By permission of the American Heart Association, Inc.)

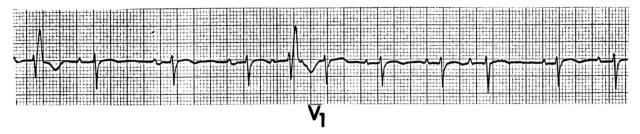

ECG III–27. *Functional aberration (PAC).* Salient features: 1. "Long-short" cycle sequence. 2. RBBB with same initial vector (r).

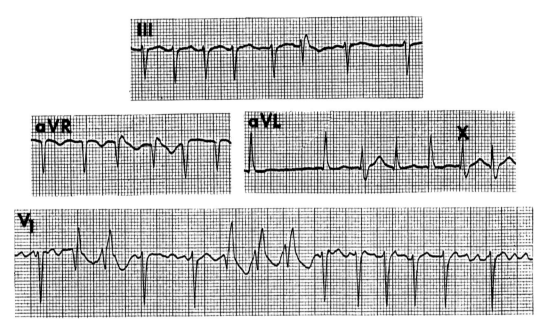

ECG III–28. *Sustained functional aberration (AF).* Salient features: 1. RBBB with same initial vector (r in III, Q in aVR, etc.) in all leads, respectively. 2. Single aberrant beats or the first aberrant beat of each multiple terminates a "long-short" sequence (although this can be minimal, as in the case of X).

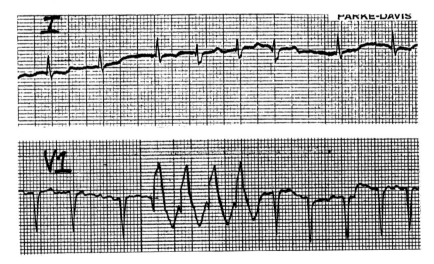

ECG III–29. *Sustained functional aberration (AF).* Salient features: 1. "Long-short" cycle sequence. 2. RBBB with same initial vector (q in I and V$_1$) in both leads, respectively.

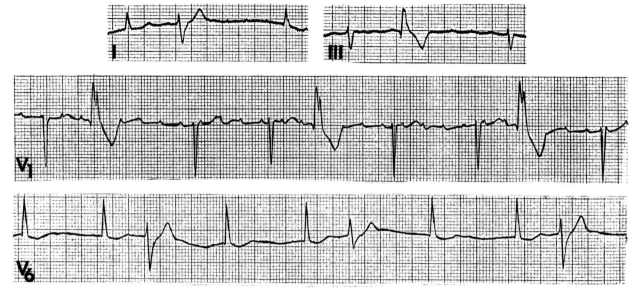

ECG III–30. *Functional aberration (AF).* Salient features: 1. "Long-short" cycle sequence. 2. RBBB; although the initial vector is different in all leads, respectively, the QRS morphology conforms to that of RBBB plus left posterior hemiblock.

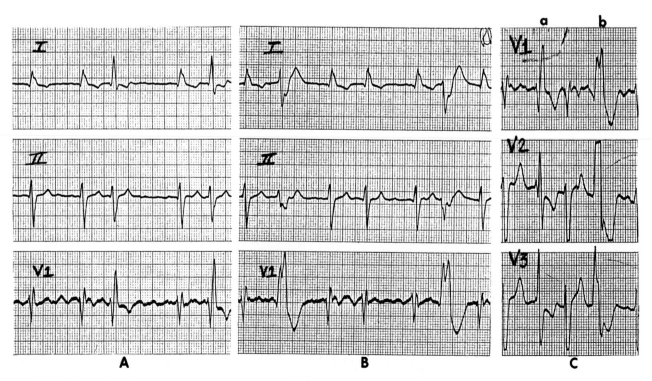

ECG III–31. *AF with both functional aberration and PVCs:* Panel A: Functional aberration. RBBB with same initial vector. (Left anterior hemiblock is present in narrow and aberrant beats). Panel B: PVCs. They do not conform to classic RBBB or RBBB plus a hemiblock; the initial vector is different. Panel C: One aberrant beat (a) and one PVC (b). Note that the PVC does not terminate a "long-short" cycle sequence.

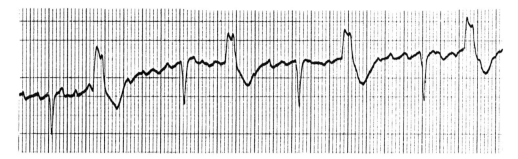

ECG III–32. *AF with PVCs.* Conducted beats have QS (or, possibly rS) morphology; the PVCs are fixed-coupled and consist of wide R-waves.

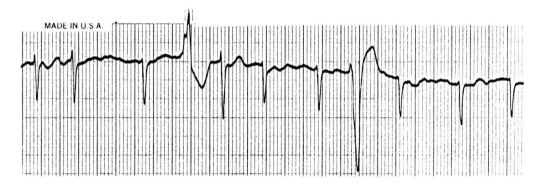

ECG III–33. *AF with multiforme PVCs.* Conducted beats are rS. PVCs are RR' and rS, respectively.

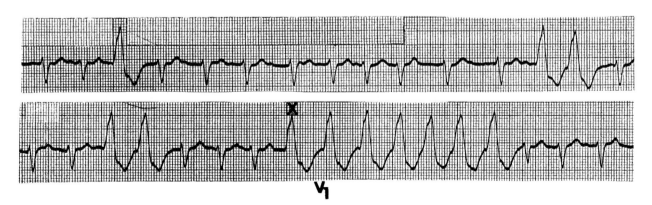

ECG III–34. *AF with a run of VT.* The conducted beats are rS. The PVCs are broad R-waves of about 0.20 sec. duration. Note the first beat of the run (X) does not terminate a "long-short" cycle sequence.

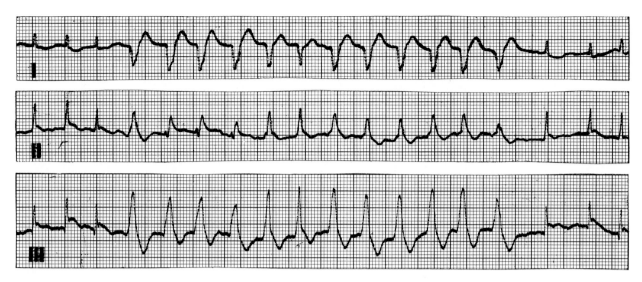

ECG III–35. *AF with a run of VT.* The wide complexes do not conform to a known bundle branch block or bifascicular pattern. The first beat of the run does not terminate a "long-short" cycle sequence.

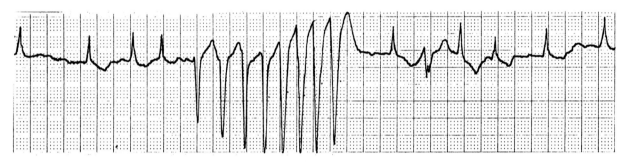

ECG III–36. *AF with a run of accelerating VT.* The run does not begin with a "long-short" cycle sequence. The cadence of the VT is greatly different (i.e., faster) than that of the underlying AF.

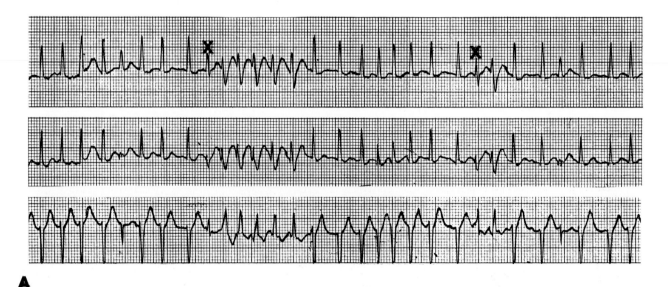

A

ECG III–37. *AF with a rapid response and both sustained functional aberration and PVCs.* A. Sustained functional aberration. The first beat (X) terminates a "long-short" cycle sequence. The morphology conforms to a classic RBBB; the initial vector is identical to that of the conducted beats in each lead. In this case, in the first beat of each sequence (X), the RBBB is only partially developed.

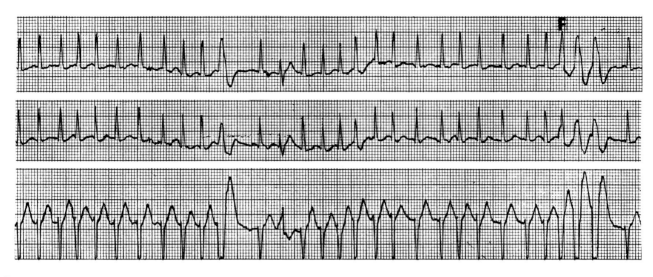

B

ECG III–37 (cont'd).   B. The PVC-triplet has LBBB morphology and begins with a fusion beat (F). The isolated PVC does not terminate a "long-short" cycle sequence. However, the "long-short" following the PVC is terminated by a functionally aberrant beat.

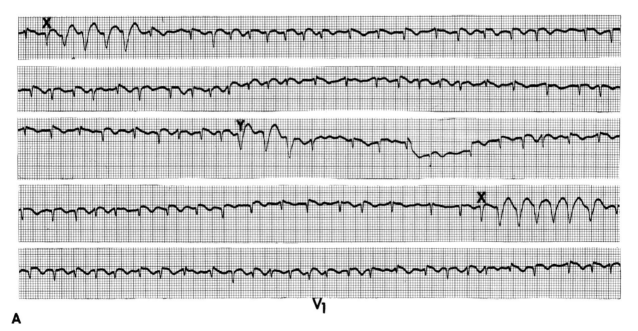

A

ECG III–38.   *AF with sustained functional aberration of LBBB-type.* A. AF with a rapid response. Runs of wide beats having LBBB morphology are present. The first beat (X) in two of the sequences shows incomplete LBBB. The first beat (Y) of the second sequence terminates a minimally "long-short" cycle sequence. Cycle sequence comparison reveals many other, more pronounced "long-short" sequences not terminated by aberrant beats. This unfavorable comparison as well as the LBBB morphology strongly suggests VT.

PROCAINAMIDE

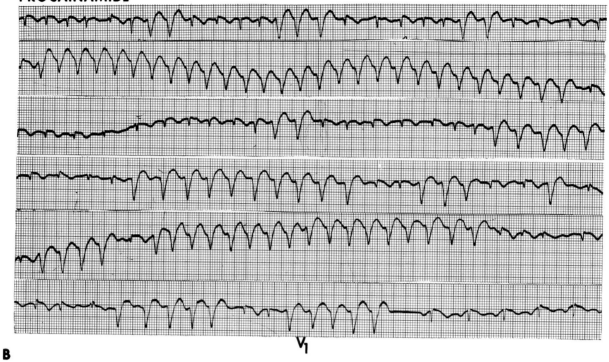

V₁

B

ECG III–38 (cont'd).   B. Following antiarrhythmic therapy with procainamide, however, the frequency and duration of the runs of wide beats greatly increase. Such a response strongly suggests sustained functional aberration. At the end of the rhythm strip, the rhythm converts to sinus.

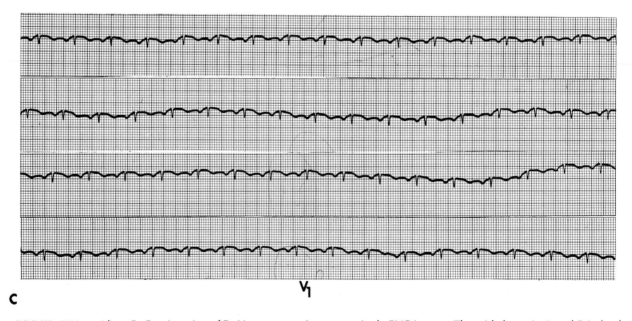

V₁

C

ECG III–38 (cont'd).   C. Continuation of B. Upon conversion, not a single PVC is seen. The wide beats in A and B indeed represented functional aberration. With the advent of sinus rhythm, elimination of R–R cycle variation put an end to the aberration.

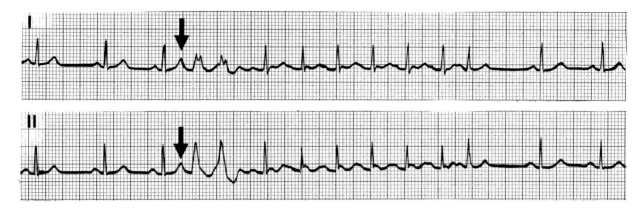

A

ECG III–39. *Continuation of a supraventricular tachyarrhythmia despite termination of sustained functional aberration.* A. Paroxysmal AF, the first two beats of which have LBBB functional aberration. The run begins with a PAC (arrow).

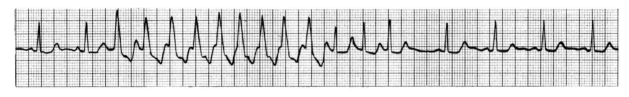

B

ECG III–39 (cont'd). B. PAT, the first nine beats of which are conducted with functional aberration.

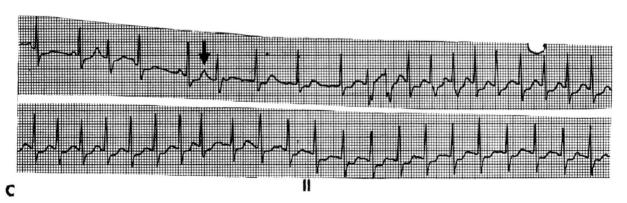

C

ECG III–39 (cont'd). C. AF beginning with a PAC (arrow). There is a five-beat run of sustained functional aberration. The first two beats have RBBB plus left anterior hemiblock; the last three have RBBB alone.

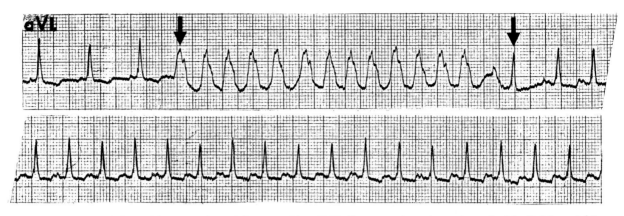

ECG III–40.   *VT followed by PAT.* The VT begins with a PVC (first arrow), and consists of wide (0.20 sec.) bizarre QRS-complexes, occurring irregularly at a rate of 190–220 bpm. During the VT, no P-waves are visible. Following the VT, there is one antegrade (perhaps sinus) capture (second arrow) followed by a run of PAT, which is regular at a rate of 137 bpm. An ectopic P-wave precedes each narrow QRS-complex. This unusual sequence of tachyarrhythmias is in contradistinction to initial sustained functional aberration of a supraventricular tachyarrhythmia, as illustrated in ECG III–39.

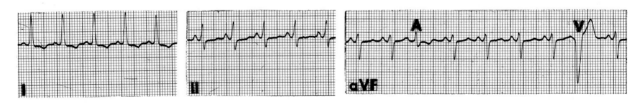

A

ECG III–41.   *PAT with runs of VT at about the same rate.* A. Baseline ECG. The basic rhythm is sinus tachycardia at 122 bpm. One PAC (A), conducted with mild functional aberration, and one PVC (V) are present.

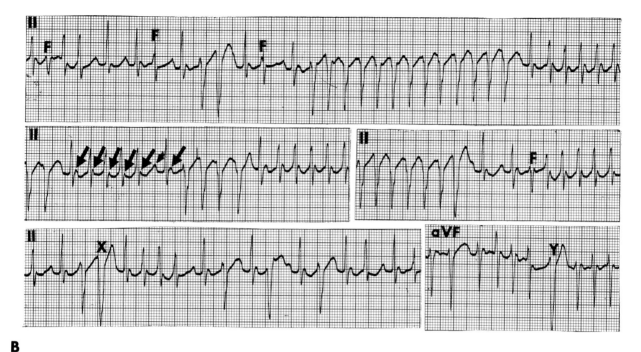

B

ECG III–41 (cont'd).   B. During PAT. The basic rhythm is PAT with close to 1:1 A–V conduction. The atrial rate is 230 bpm. Arrows point to several adjacent P-waves. There are frequent PVCs, as well as couplets, triplets, and short runs of VT. The VT is slightly irregular; the average rate is also 230 bpm. That these are not merely supraventricular beats with functional aberration is proven by (1) their resemblance to the PVC (V) in the baseline ECG, (2) the presence of fusion beats (F)*, and (3) the lack of a "long-short" cycle sequence preceding one of the beats (Y).

---

*Actually, most of the PVCs are in some degree of fusion, since the supraventricular beats almost simultaneously occur. One of the more "pure" PVCs is labeled X.

PROPRANOLOL

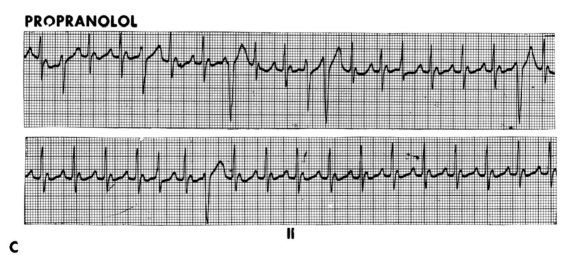

C

ECG III–41 (cont'd).   C. After intravenous propranolol, A–V conduction decreases essentially to 2:1. PVCs are still present, although the runs of VT are suppressed.

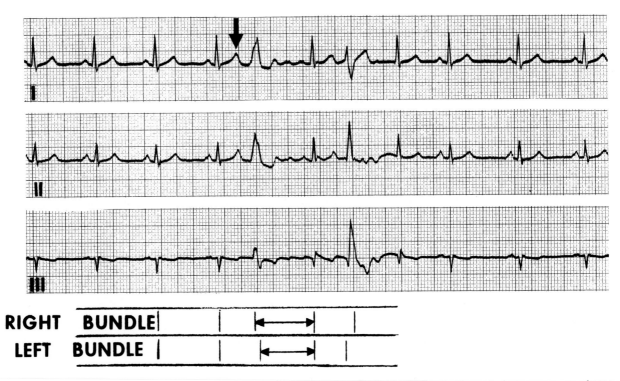

ECG III–42. *Bigeminal functional aberration with alternating BBB.* The basic rhythm is sinus. A short paroxysm of AF is triggered by a PAC (arrow). The PAC is conducted with functional aberration of LBBB-type. Following this beat, during AF, another "long-short" cycle sequence is terminated by a beat conducted with functional aberration of RBBB-type. This bigeminal functional aberration with alternating BBB is seen most often during sinus rhythm with PACs in bigeminy. The mechanism of this alternation is shown in the diagram. During the first aberrant beat (LBBB), conduction in the left bundle branch is delayed. The long cycle of the "long-short" cycle sequence preceding the second aberrant beat is therefore longer for the right bundle than for the left. Thus the aberration of the second beat is of RBBB-type.

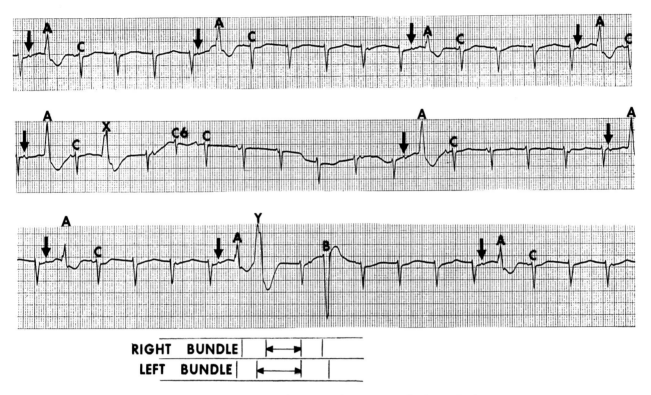

ECG III–43. *Functional aberration during incomplete A–V dissociation.* The basic rhythm is an accelerated junctional rhythm at 93 bpm. The underlying sinus rate is somewhat slower, about 84 bpm. Obvious periods of A–V dissociation are present. There are a number of early narrow QRSs (C). Since each is preceded by a sinus-P-wave, these beats represent sinus captures. Note that in the case of C6, the P-wave occurs at the tail-end of the preceding junctional QRS; we now have the important information that such an early P-wave can capture, albeit with a long P–R interval. (Incomplete) A–V dissociation is present because the junctional rate exceeds the rate of the sinus; A–V block is not present. Two obvious PVCs (X and Y) are present. Each is a wide QRS-complex not preceded by a P-wave.

What are the beats labeled "A"? These are wide QRS-complexes having a RBBB morphology. Although they resemble the PVC labeled "X," each "A" beat is preceded by a sinus-P-wave (arrow); we know from C6 that all of these P-waves could capture. Are the "A" beats PVCs or captures with functional aberration of RBBB-type? The answer is contained in the "A-Y-B" series of beats in the bottom strip, and the accompanying diagram.

"Y" is a PVC having a morphology akin to RBBB. The PVC therefore arises in the left ventricle. As the electrical impulse spreads through the myocardium, it encounters the left bundle before encountering the right bundle. Let us now turn to B. It has a LBBB morphology and is preceded by a sinus-P-wave. It also terminates a "long-short" cycle sequence. The long cycle of the "long-short" is longer for the left bundle than for the right. If B were a conducted beat with functional aberration, it would therefore have a LBBB morphology. Indeed, B has the configuration of LBBB! Given the specific circumstances created by the preceding PVC, it is too coincidental for B to be a PVC. The captures terminating "long-short" cycle sequences are therefore conducted with functional aberration. This is ordinarily RBBB (i.e., the "A" beats), except when the preceding long cycle is longer for the left bundle (i.e., B). C6, although also terminating a "long-short" cycle sequence heralded by a PVC, does not have functional aberration, presumably because its preceding short cycle is slightly longer than the short cycle immediately preceding B.

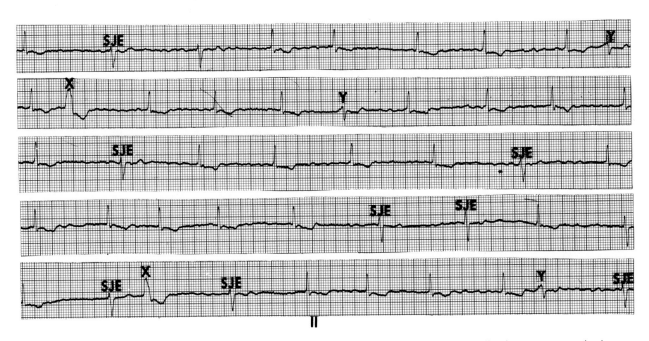

ECG III–44 (Lead II; Leads V₁, V₂ and V₆ on next page).   *Atrial fibrillation with a generally slow response.* The longest R–R intervals are equal; the QRS-complexes terminating such R–R intervals have a RBBB + left anterior hemiblock pattern, and, therefore, represent subjunctional escape beats (SJE) arising from the posterior division of the left bundle. Note that the SJE rate is not accelerated (41/min.). The patient is well digitalized. Note the wide premature beats—those having a LBBB/normal axis pattern (X), and those with a LBBB/left axis pattern (Y). On the surface they would appear to be PVCs, since a LBBB pattern is unusual with functional aberration. However, note that in the bottom strip of Lead II, as well as in the V leads, they are followed by SJEs. If one sets one's calipers for the true SJE time (e.g., the R–R interval between the two SJEs in the fourth strip of Lead II), and goes back one cycle-length from the SJE following X and Y beats, one finds that the subjunctional pacemaker has been reset from *in front of* the X and Y QRSs. This indicates that X and Y are really supraventricular beats (i.e., an atrial fibrillation impulse must have antegradely traversed the subjunctional pacemaker site and reset it); LBBB functional aberration is present.

To summarize, in this case of atrial fibrillation, functional aberration was differentiated from PVCs on the basis of the reset point of a subsequent (sub) junctional escape beat. If these are really supraventricular beats with functional aberration, the (sub) junction would be traversed *antegradely*, at some point *in front of* the QRS. If truly PVCs, the (sub) junction would be traversed *retrogradely*, at some point *following* the QRS.

Of additional interest, note that the Y-beat in the second strip of Lead II is only slightly premature yet still shows functional aberration. This is presumably because there has been concealed penetration of the proximal bundle branches by one of the atrial fibrillation impulses at some point between the preceding QRS and Y. The true "short" cycle of the "long-short" cycle sequence required for functional aberration is indeed short, and Y in this strip represents the *second* beat of sustained functional aberration.

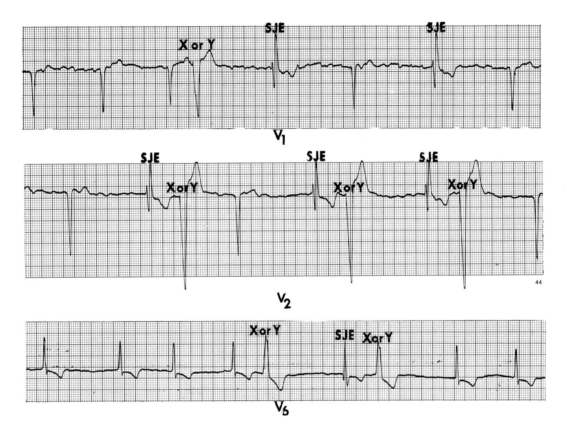

ECG III–44 (cont'd).

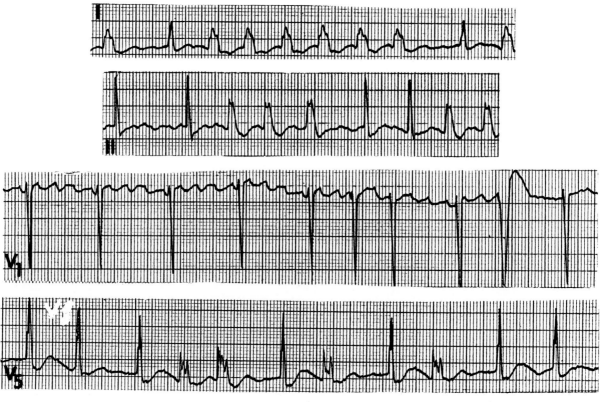

A

ECG III–45. *Three types of intermittent (left) BBB in AF.* A. Sustained functional aberration. The aberrant beats begin with a "long-short" cycle sequence. The aberration, once begun, disappears when the rate slows.

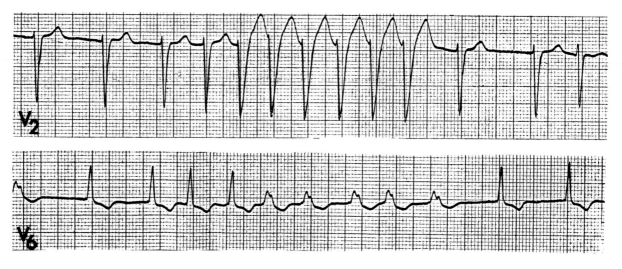

B

ECG III–45 (cont'd). B. Rate-related BBB. The aberration occurs at faster rates, but not always with a significant "long-short" cycle sequence. Occasionally, it takes one or more beats for the aberration to appear when the rate increases above the critical point, and/or one or more beats for the aberration to disappear when the rate slows below the critical point ("fatigue").

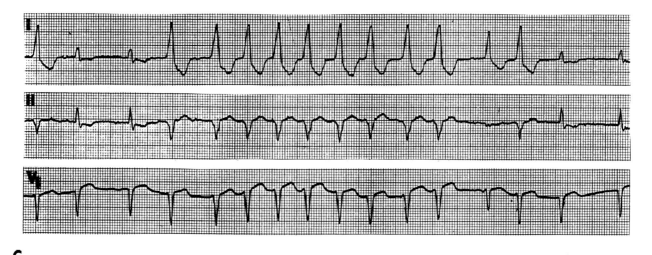

C

ECG III–45 (cont'd).   C. Random-intermittent BBB. The aberration appears randomly, and is not related to rate or "long-short" cycle sequences.

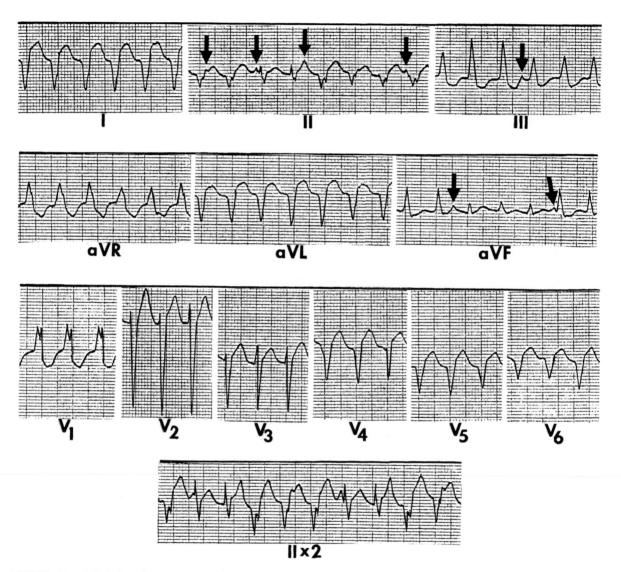

ECG III–46.   *VT. Salient features:* 1. Tachycardia with wide QRS at 150 bpm. 2. QRSs do not conform to known fascicular pattern (i.e., marked right axis [+150°] with QS in I; R in V_1 and QS in V_6). 3. Identifiable periods of A–V dissociation. Arrows indicate identifiable P-waves; these have no relationship to the QRSs. QRS morphology variation in Leads II, III and aVF is secondary to respiratory effect, and not sinus captures or fusion beats, since these QRS changes occur regardless of the presence or absence of P-waves preceding them.

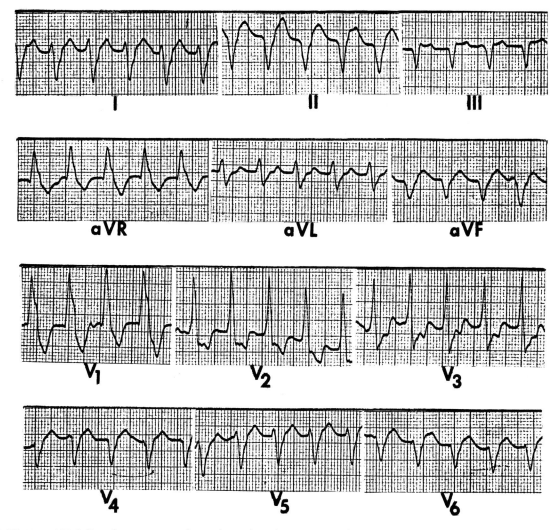

ECG III–47. *VT. Salient features:* 1. Tachycardia with wide QRS at 125 bpm. 2. QRSs do not conform to known fascicular pattern (i.e., "northwest" axis of −120°; rS in I and QS in II, III, and aVF; qR in V_1 and rS in V_6).

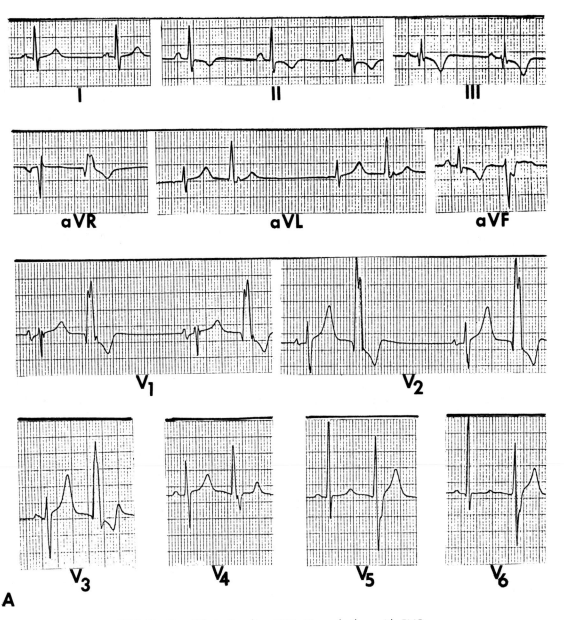

ECG III–48. *VT.* A. Baseline ECG. Sinus rhythm with PVCs.

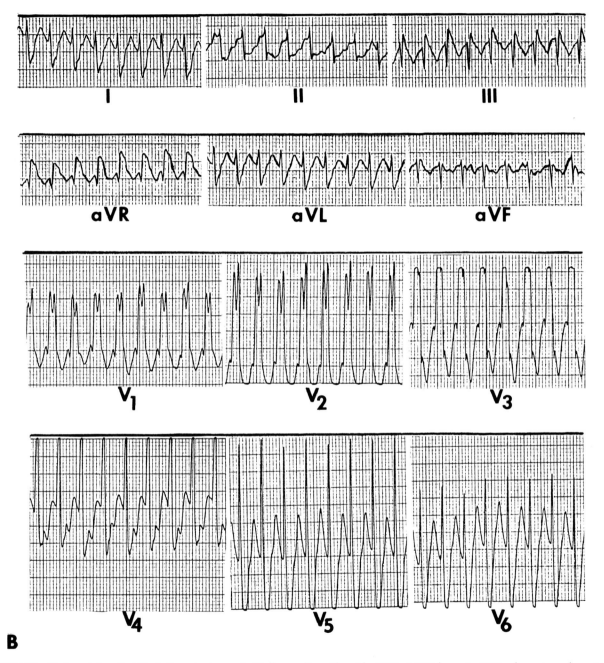

B

ECG III–48 (cont'd). B. VT. Salient features: 1. Tachycardia with wide QRS at 215 bpm 2. QRSs do not conform to known bifascicular pattern (i.e., "northwest" axis of −120°; rS in I and rSr' in aVF). 3. Morphology of QRSs matches the PVC morphology in the baseline ECG.

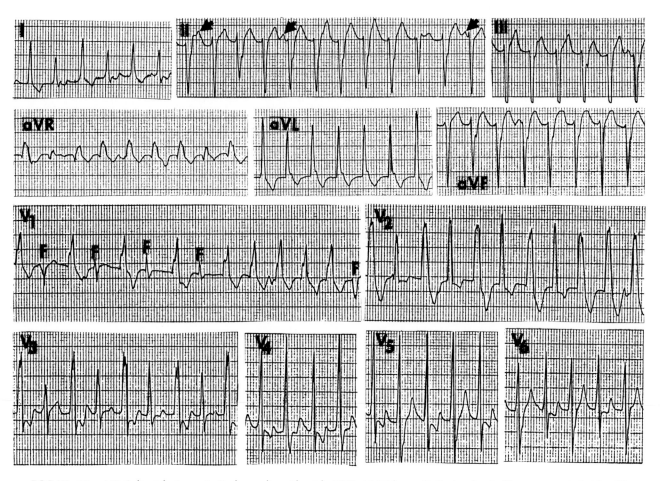

ECG III–49.   *VT. Salient features:* 1. Tachycardia with wide QRS at 165 bpm. 2. Fusion beats (F) are present. 3. Identifiable P-waves (arrows) with A–V dissociation are present (see Lead II).

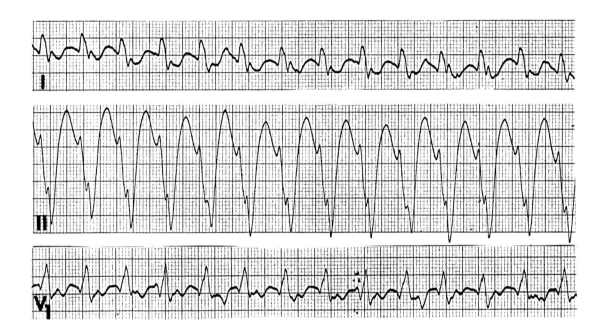

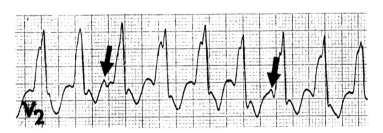

ECG III–50. *VT. Salient features:* 1. Tachycardia with wide QRS at 122 bpm. 2. Exceptionally wide QRSs (0.26 sec.). 3. Identifiable P-waves (arrows) with A–V dissociation.

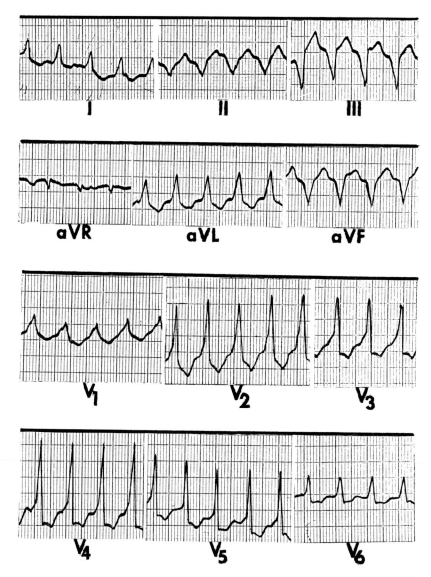

ECG III–51. *VT. Salient features:* 1. Tachycardia with wide QRS at 150 bpm. 2. Unusual precordial morphology (R in V$_1$ and R in V$_6$). (Stein, E. *The Electrocardiogram: A Self-Study Course in Clinical Electrocardiography.* Courtesy of W. B. Saunders Co., 1976.)

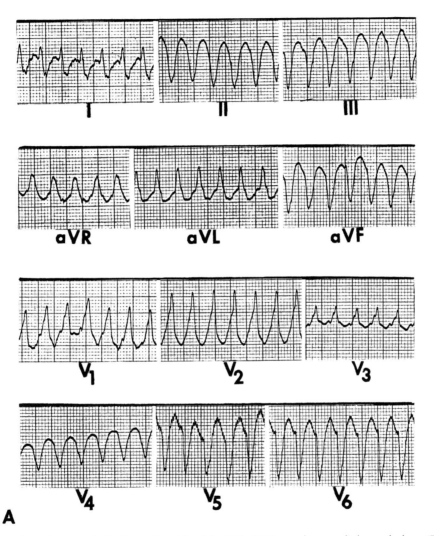

ECG III–52. *VT. Salient features:* 1. Tachycardia with wide QRS. 2. Unusual precordial morphology (R in V_1 and QS in V_6). A. Rate 215 bpm.

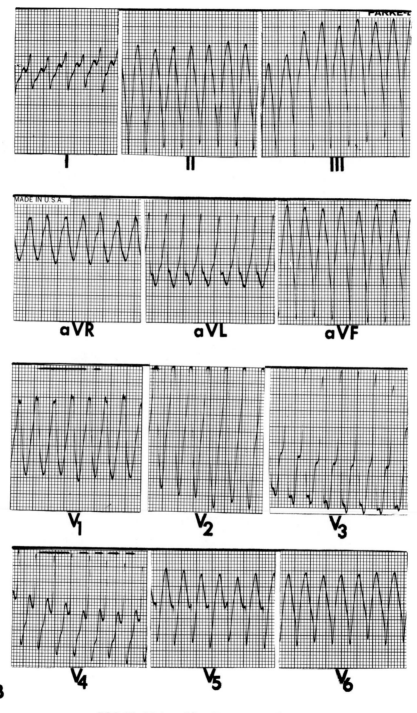

ECG III–52 (cont'd).   B. Rate 263 bpm.

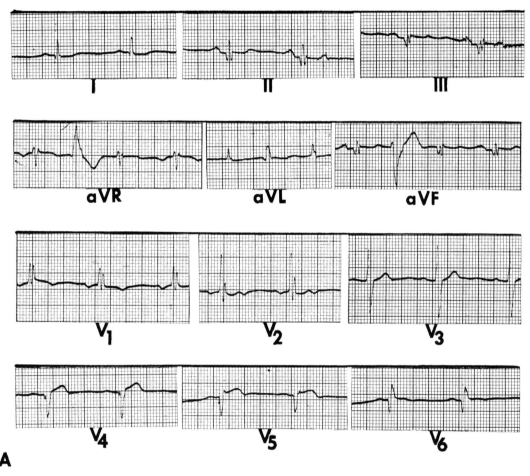

ECG III–53. *VT.* A. Baseline ECG. There are extensive inferodorsal and anterolateral myocardial infarctions. Note the PVCs (aVR, aVL, aVF).

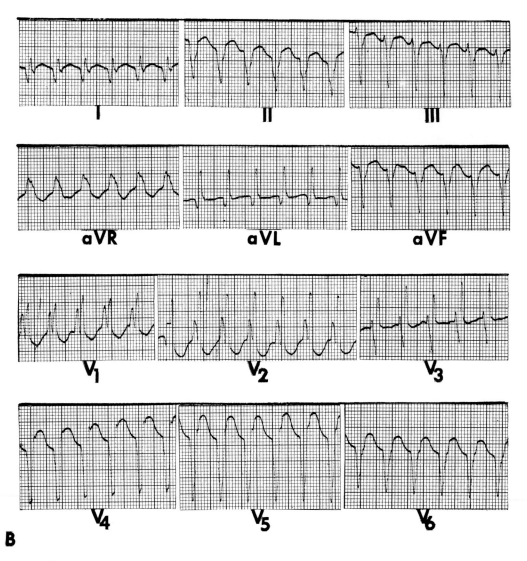

B

ECG III–53 (cont'd).   B. VT. Salient features: 1. Tachycardia with wide QRS at 166 bpm. 2. QRS morphology is bizarre. Although the initial vectors match the initial vectors of the sinus beats in the precordial leads, there is a discordance in the following frontal leads:

	Sinus beat	VT
I	q (rapid, small)	Q (large, slurred)
III	Q	r
aVR	r (rapid, small)	R (large, slurred)
aVL	R	Q

Note also the resemblance of the VT to the PVCs in the baseline ECG.

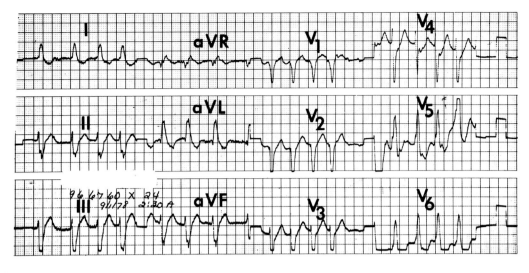

A

ECG III–54. *VT in AF with both left and right BBB.* A. Baseline ECG 9/1. AF with LBBB.

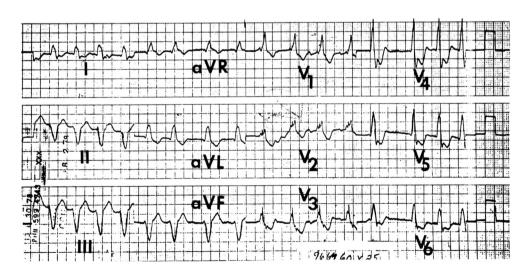

B

ECG III–54 (cont'd). B. Baseline ECG 9/2. AF with RBBB and left anterior hemiblock.

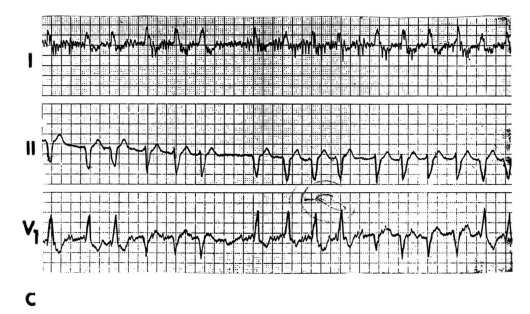

C

ECG III–54 (cont'd).   C. Baseline ECG 10/6. AF with both LBBB and RBBB (plus left anterior hemiblock).

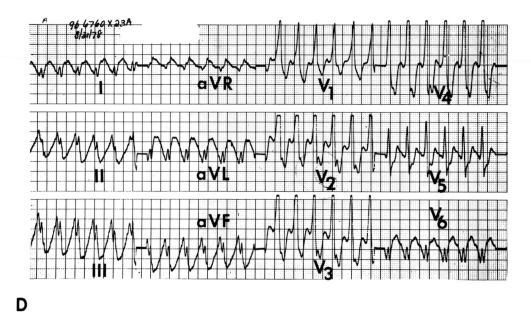

D

ECG III–54 (cont'd).   D. VT. The QRS-complexes are bizarre, and do not conform to either BBB pattern (i.e., notched QS in I and V$_6$). The rhythm is regular at 160 bpm.

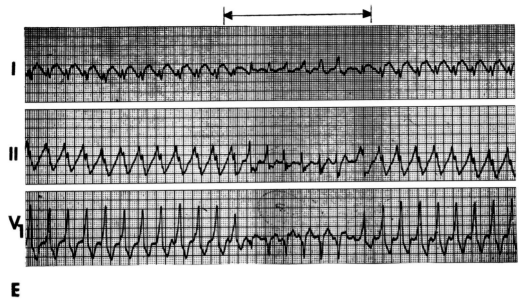

ECG III–54 (cont'd). E. Rhythm strip during VT. A series of fusion beats (bracket) occur.

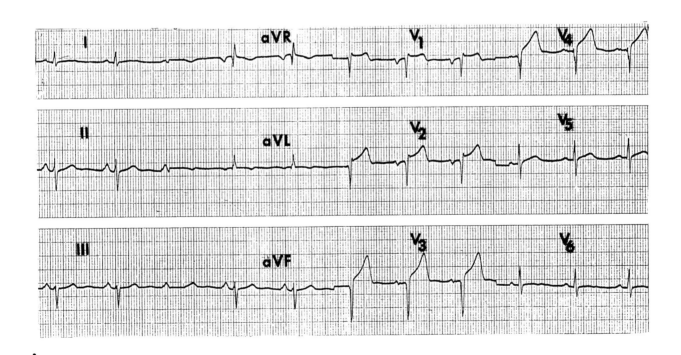

ECG III–55. *VT with 1:1 V–A conduction.* A. Baseline ECG. The rhythm is sinus. There is an acute anteroseptal MI and left anterior hemiblock.

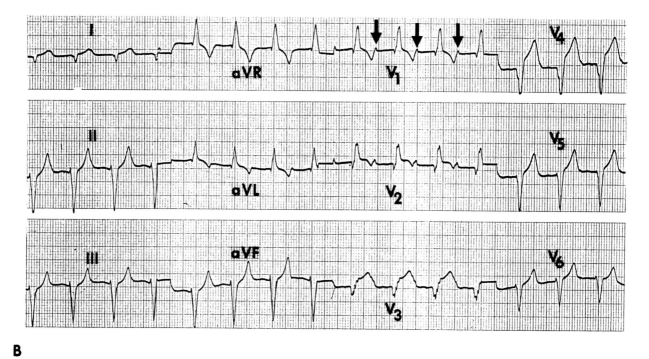

B

ECG III–55 (cont'd).   B. VT. The QRS-complexes are wide and bizarre ("northwest" axis with QS in I, qR in V₁, and rS in V₆). The initial vector in Lead I (QS) is different than the initial vector in Lead I of the baseline ECG (qR). The rhythm is thus established as ventricular in origin. P-waves (arrows) are visible in Leads V₁ and V₂. They are retrograde-P-waves (i.e., 1:1 V–A conduction), since they are related in constant fashion to the QRSs. (Remember that retrograde-P-waves are usually upright in those leads.) The rate of 100 bpm is at the lower limit for VT.

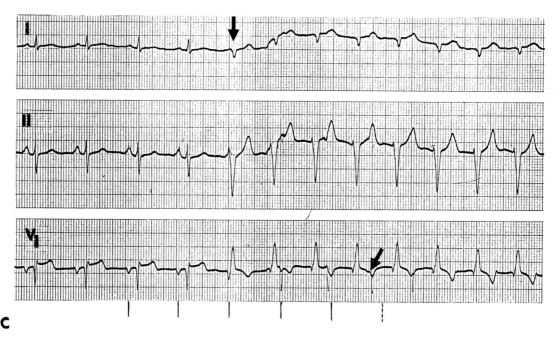

C

ECG III–55 (cont'd).   C. Onset of VT. The VT begins with a PVC (first arrow). During the first three beats, A–V dissociation is present. The fourth beat is followed by a retrograde-P-wave (second arrow). This comes earlier than the expected sinus-P-wave (broken line). The R–P interval (i.e., V–A conduction time) then progressively increases.

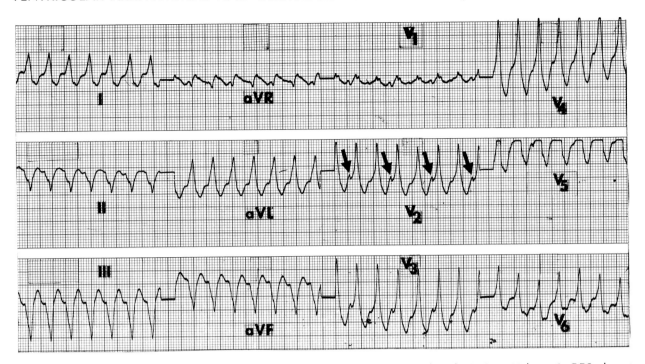

ECG III–56. *VT with 2:1 V–A conduction.* Salient features: 1. Tachycardia with wide QRS at 190 bpm. 2. QRSs do not conform to known fascicular pattern (i.e., R in V_1 and V_6). 3. Upright P-waves are clearly identifiable in Lead V_2, and are related to every other QRS in constant fashion. These P-waves (arrows) are therefore retrograde-P-waves, and represent 2:1 V–A conduction.

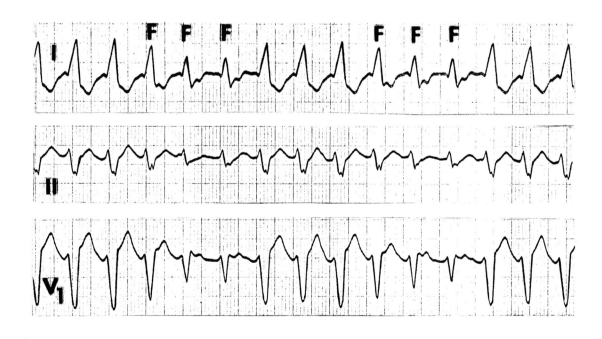

A

ECG III–57. *VT with fusion beats (F).* A. The rate is 144 bpm.

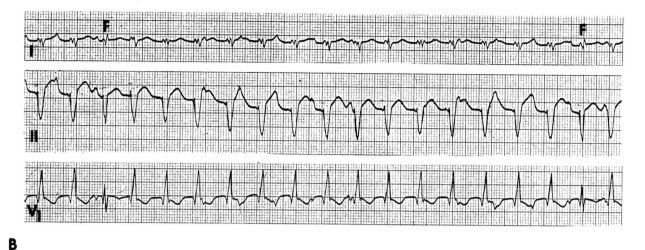

B

ECG III–57 (cont'd).   B. The rate is slightly irregular at about 115 bpm. A–V dissociation is present. In addition to the P-waves preceding the fusion beats, can you spot the other identifiable P-waves?

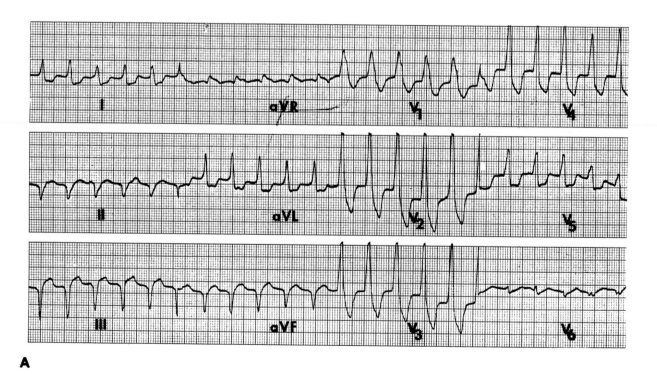

A

ECG III–58.   *VT.* A. Patient was admitted to the hospital because of mild congestive heart failure. Admission ECG revealed a wide-QRS tachycardia at 135 bpm. A telephone report of an ECG taken during an earlier hospitalization at a different hospital stated that a RBBB had been present. What is the diagnosis?

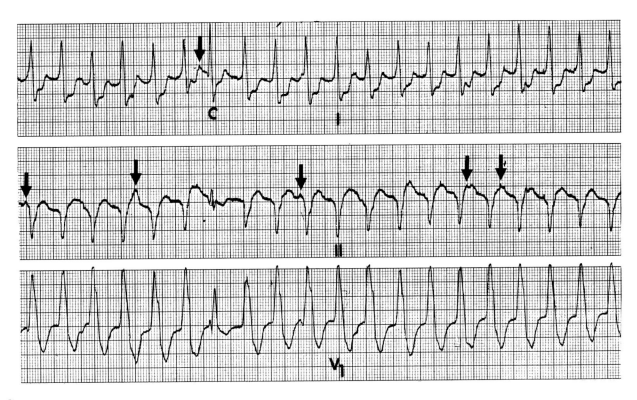

B

ECG III–58 (cont'd).   B. Examination of a long rhythm strip reveals A–V dissociation. Some of the visible P-waves are marked by arrows. The differential diagnosis is between accelerated junctional/subjunctional rhythm and VT. One early beat (C) occurs. Since it is preceded by a P-wave which could have captured, it is presumably a sinus capture. Note that the morphology of the capture is different than that of the dominant rhythm, and consists of a classic RBBB pattern (qRs in I, rsR' in V₁). The dominant rhythm is, therefore, VT. Note that Lead II reveals an inferior wall MI.

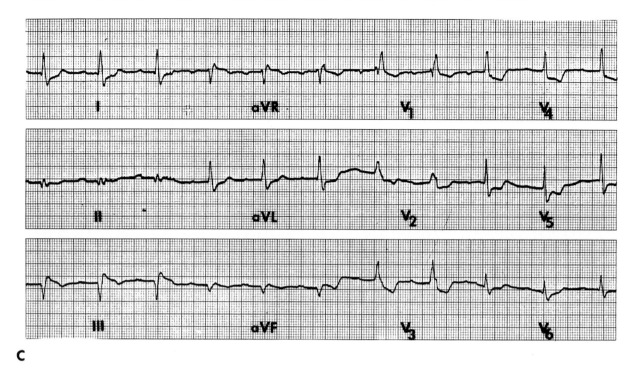

C

ECG III–58 (cont'd).   C. Following conversion to sinus rhythm the QRS morphology is identical to the morphology of the single capture during VT.

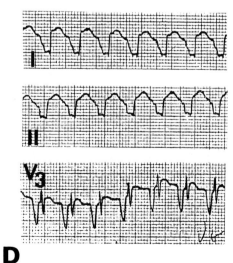

ECG III–58 (cont'd).   D. *VT masquerading as PAT* (in another patient). The QRS morphology in Lead V₃ gives the illusion of large P-waves followed by narrow QRSs.

D

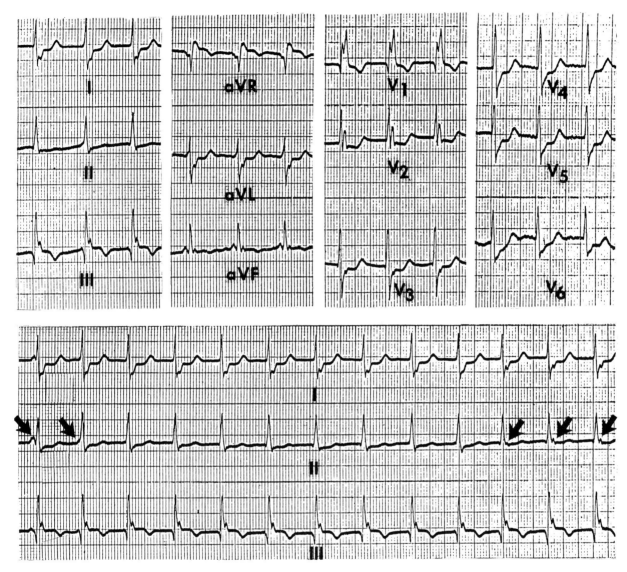

ECG III–59. *Accelerated junctional/subjunctional rhythm.* In this 3-channel recording there is a regular rhythm at 97/min. The QRS morphology is that of typical RBBB. Sinus-P-waves at a rate of 94/min. are visible in Lead aVF, and appear to conduct with a short P–R interval. However, inspection of the long rhythm strip reveals complete A–V dissociation, with the P-waves (arrows) merging into the QRS-complexes at the beginning of the strip (note the abolition of the initial Q-wave in Leads II and III in the first few beats), and re-emerging from the QRS-complexes by the end of the strip (note the abolition of the S-wave in Lead II in the last few beats). Since the QRS morphology conforms to a known RBBB pattern, the beats originate from either the junction (accelerated junctional rhythm with RBBB) or the left bundle (accelerated subjunctional rhythm). The finding of normal QRS-complexes in either a previous ECG or in sinus captures in the present ECG would suggest the latter. Sinus captures are not present in the tracing provided, but since no P-waves occur in a position to capture, *the presence of A–V block cannot be ascertained.*

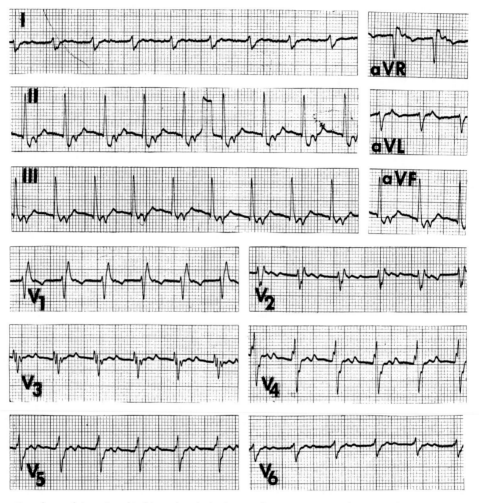

ECG III–60. *Accelerated junctional/subjunctional rhythm with 1:1 V–A conduction.* The rate is 84 bpm. The QRS morphology is that of typical RBBB. A retrograde-P-wave follows each QRS.

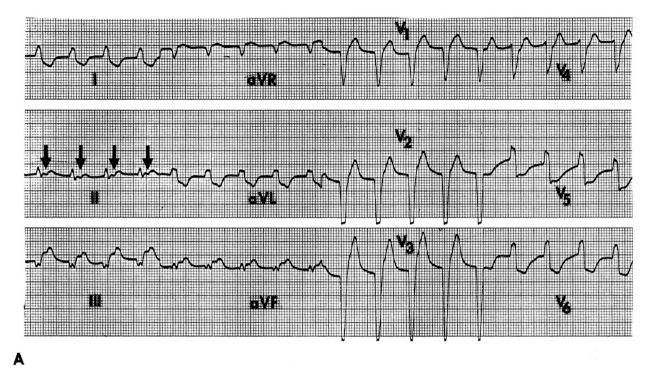

A

ECG III–61. *Accelerated junctional rhythm with LBBB.* The rate is 115 bpm. A. There is a wide-QRS tachycardia with a LBBB morphology. A retrograde-P-wave (arrows) follows each QRS. The differential diagnosis is between VT and accelerated junctional/subjunctional rhythm.

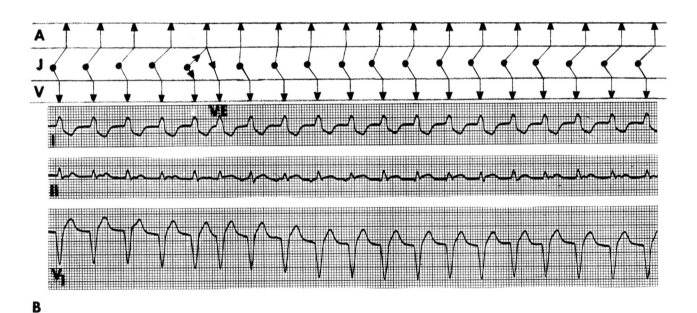

B

ECG III–61 (cont'd).   B. At the beginning of the rhythm strip, the R–P intervals lengthen (see Lead II). This V–A Wencke-bach period culminates in a *ventricular echo* (VE). The ventricular echo has the same LBBB morphology as the dominant rhythm. Since the ventricular echo is a supraventricular beat, the LBBB must have preexisted, and the dominant rhythm must also be supraventricular (i.e., accelerated junctional) with LBBB. Following the ventricular echo, another long V–A Wencke-bach period unfolds.

A = Atria; J = Junction; V = Ventricles

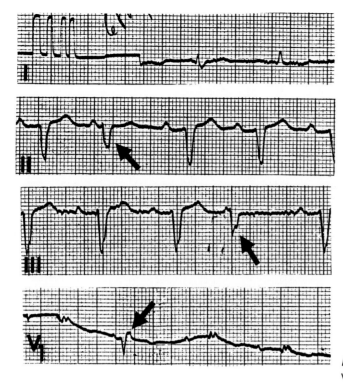

A

ECG III–62. *Accelerated junctional rhythm with RBBB and PVCs.* A. Baseline ECG. The rhythm is sinus with first-degree A–V block and RBBB. Several PVCs (arrows) are present.

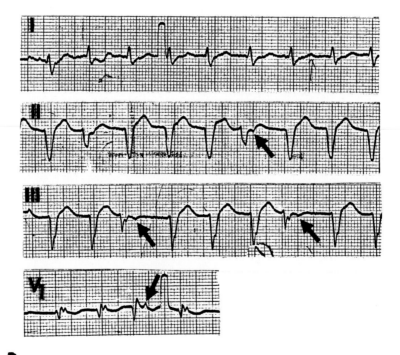

B

ECG III–62 (cont'd).   B. Accelerated junctional rhythm. There is a wide-QRS tachycardia at 115 bpm. The QRS morphology (RBBB) is identical to the morphology of the sinus beats in the baseline ECG. Several PVCs are present; the morphology is identical to the PVC morphology in the baseline ECG. Each PVC is followed by a retrograde-P-wave (arrows).

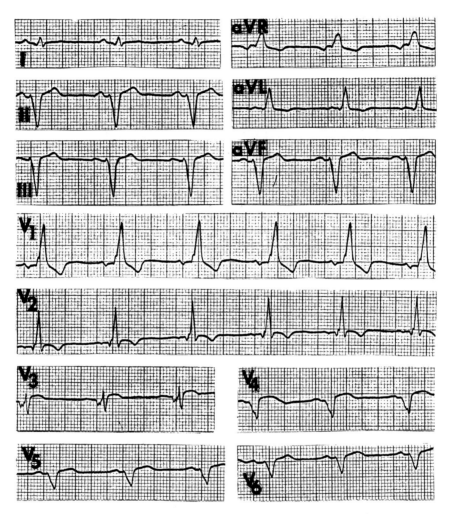

ECG III–63. Twelve-lead ECG showing sinus rhythm with extensive anterolateral myocardial infarction, complete RBBB and left anterior hemiblock. There is a qRs in I, R in V_1, and QS in V_6. With such bizarre morphology, a supraventricular tachycardia could easily be mistaken for VT, if the baseline ECG were not available.

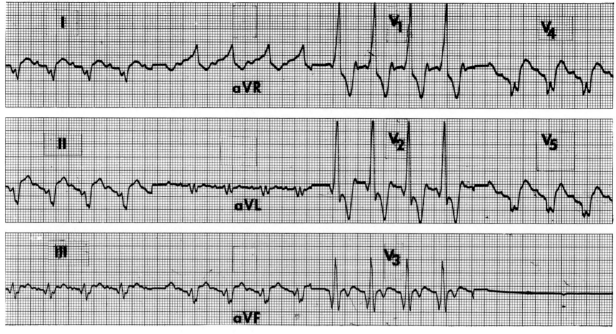

A

ECG III–64. *Accelerated junctional rhythm with bizarre QRS.* A. Baseline ECG. Patient is hyperkalemic and on procainamide. The rhythm is sinus. The QRSs are markedly wide (0.18 sec.) and bizarre, reflecting hyperkalemia-induced RBBB and extensive anterior, inferior, and lateral infarctions. (Lead V₆ was not recorded.)

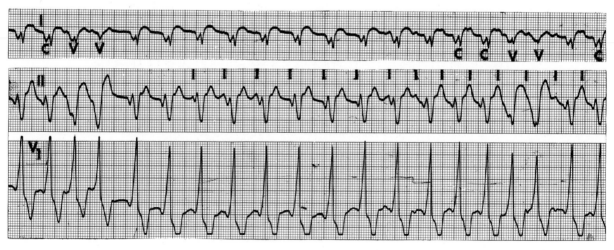

B

ECG III–64 (cont'd). B. *Accelerated junctional rhythm with PVCs.* Patient is on dopamine. There is a wide-QRS tachycardia at 110 bpm. Although the QRS morphology is bizarre, it is identical to the morphology of the sinus beats in the baseline ECG. The underlying sinus rate is 110–130 bpm. Incomplete A–V dissociation is present. Four sinus captures (early supraventricular QRSs labeled "C") are present. Two PVC couplets (V) are also present.

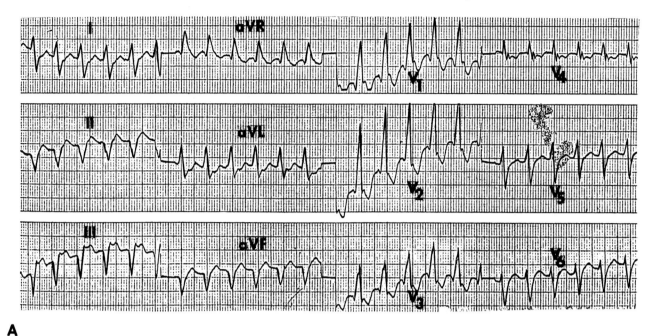

A

ECG III–65. *PAT with RBBB and left anterior hemiblock.* A. There is a wide-QRS tachycardia at 158 bpm. The QRS morphology could reflect either (1) supraventricular tachycardia with RBBB, left anterior hemiblock, and an anteroseptal MI, or (2) VT. No clear-cut P-waves are identifiable.

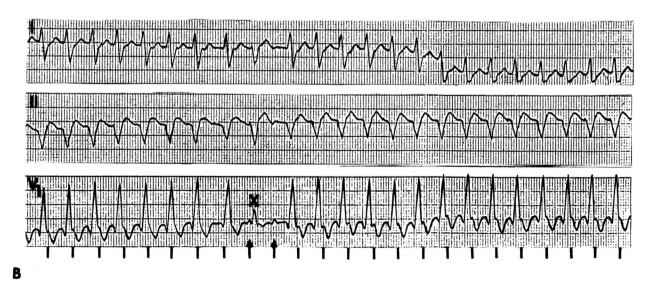

B

ECG III–65 (cont'd). B. One PVC (X) occurs. The PVC exposes two P-waves (arrows). To the right of the PVC, the P-waves have a constant relationship to the QRSs. A–V conduction is 1:1 with first-degree A–V block. The atrial rate indicates PAT at 150 bpm. To the left of the PVC, there is an A–V Wenckebach period; this is terminated by the PVC.

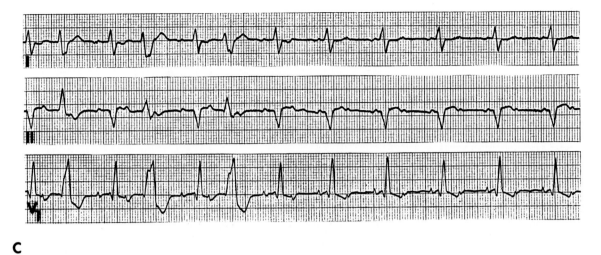

C

ECG III–65 (cont'd).   C. After digitalization, A–V conduction decreases to 2:1. Three PVCs are present.

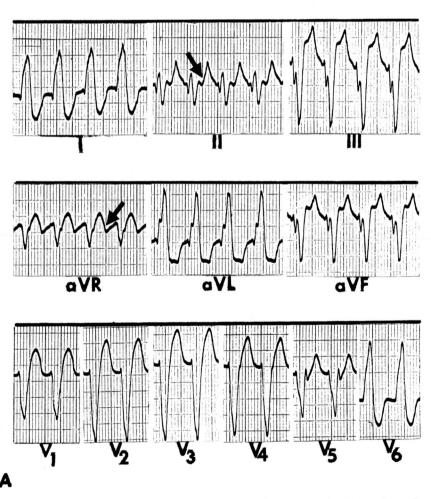

A

ECG III–66.   *Atrial flutter with 2:1 A–V conduction and LBBB.* A. There is a wide-QRS tachycardia at 144 bpm. The QRS morphology is that of LBBB. The differential diagnosis consists of (1) supraventricular tachycardia with LBBB, and (2) VT. The angularity of the baseline (arrows) suggests atrial flutter.

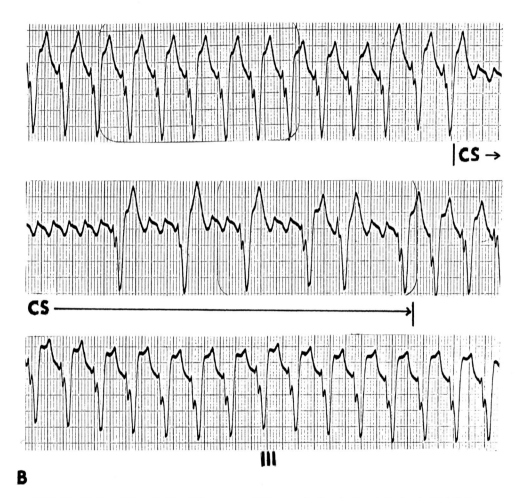

B

ECG III–66 (cont'd). B. Carotid massage (CS) reveals the rhythm is indeed atrial flutter.

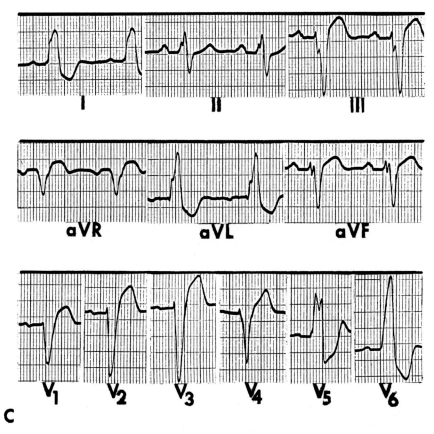

C

ECG III–66 (cont'd).   C. The previous ECG (sinus rhythm) also reveals LBBB. (Stein, E. *The Electrocardiogram: A Self-Study Course in Clinical Electrocardiography.* Courtesy of W. B. Saunders Co., 1976.)

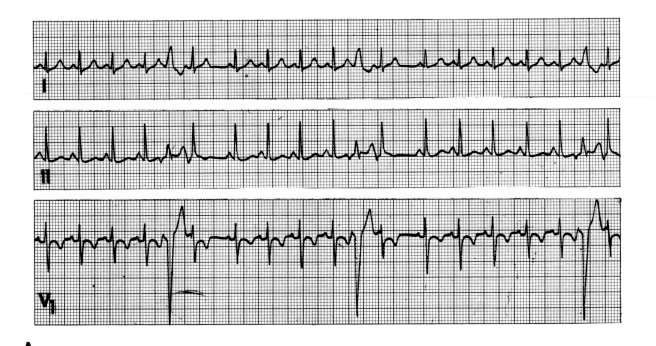

A

ECG III–67.   *Reentrant SVT (RSVT) with LBBB sustained functional aberration.* A. Baseline ECG. The basic rhythm is sinus tachycardia. There are three PAC couplets. The first PAC in each pair has functional aberration of LBBB-type.

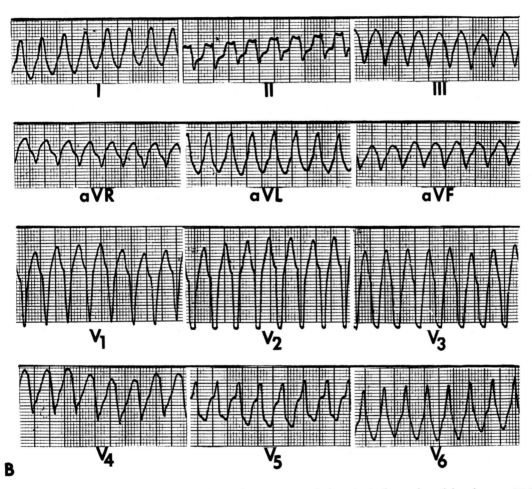

ECG III–67 (cont'd). B. RSVT. The rate is 214 bpm; the LBBB-morphology is similar to that of the aberrant PACs in the baseline ECG, except that left axis deviation is now present as well. No P-waves are visible.

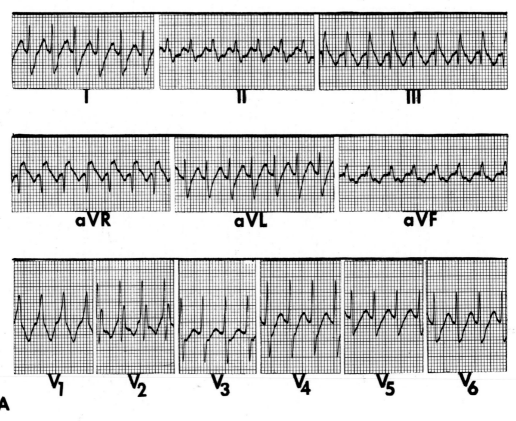

ECG III–68. *RSVT with RBBB sustained functional aberration.* A. The rate is 200 bpm. The QRS morphology is that of typical RBBB. No P-waves are visible.

B

ECG III–68 (cont'd). B. Post-digitalization. The rhythm has converted to sinus. The RBBB is no longer present.

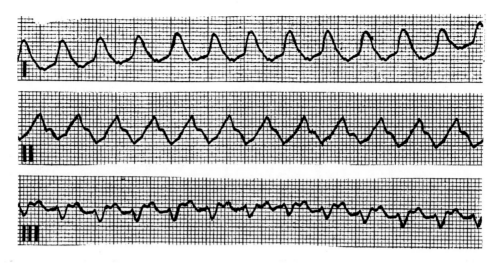

A

ECG III–69. *Atrial flutter with 2:1 A–V conduction and QRS-complexes widened by LBBB plus hyperkalemia.* A. Acidotic patient. The rate is 150 bpm. The QRSs are extremely wide (0.18 sec.) and have LBBB morphology.

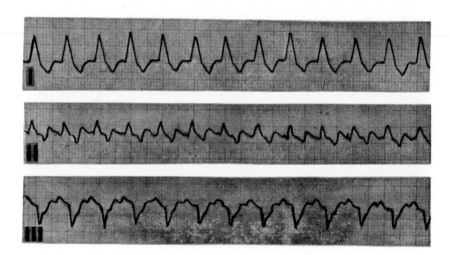

B

ECG III–69 (cont'd).   B. After sodium bicarbonate. The QRS-complexes have narrowed to 0.13 sec., but still have LBBB morphology. The flutter waves are now apparent.

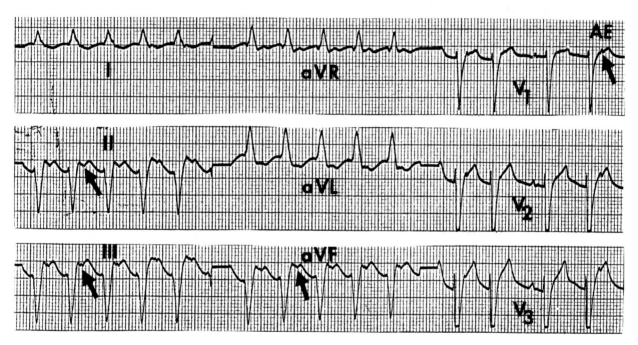

ECG III–70. *RSVT with LBBB.* In Leads I through aVF there is a wide-QRS tachycardia at 140 bpm. Retrograde-P-waves follow each QRS. These are apparent in Leads II, III, and aVF (arrows). Following the sinus beat, a PAC with first-degree A–V block triggers an atrial echo (AE). Since the sinus beat also has a LBBB, the tachyarrhythmia is a RSVT with LBBB rather than VT. The atrial echo is, of course, the beginning of a RSVT.

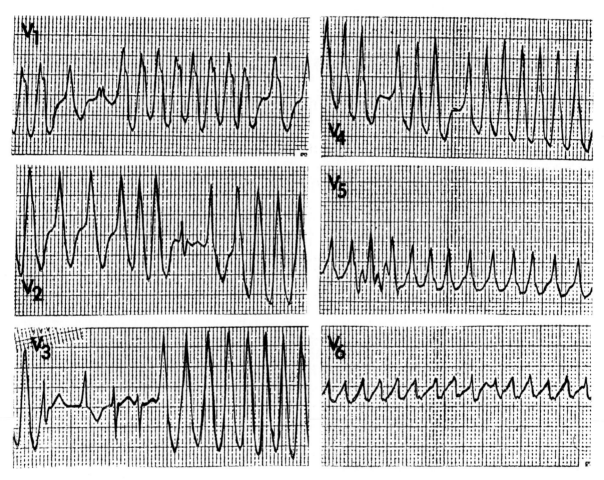

ECG III–71.   *AF with rapid Kent bundle conduction (W-P-W).* The cadence is grossly irregularly irregular. Most of the QRSs are wide and bizarre (R in V_1 and V_6). These beats represent pure antegrade Kent bundle conduction. The narrow beats represent pure A–V nodal conduction and indicate transient failure of Kent bundle conduction. Several A–V nodal-Kent fusion beats are present. At times the heart rate exceeds 300 bpm. (Reproduced with permission from Childers, R.: Classification of cardiac dysrhythmias. Med. Clin. North Am., *60:3,* 1976.)

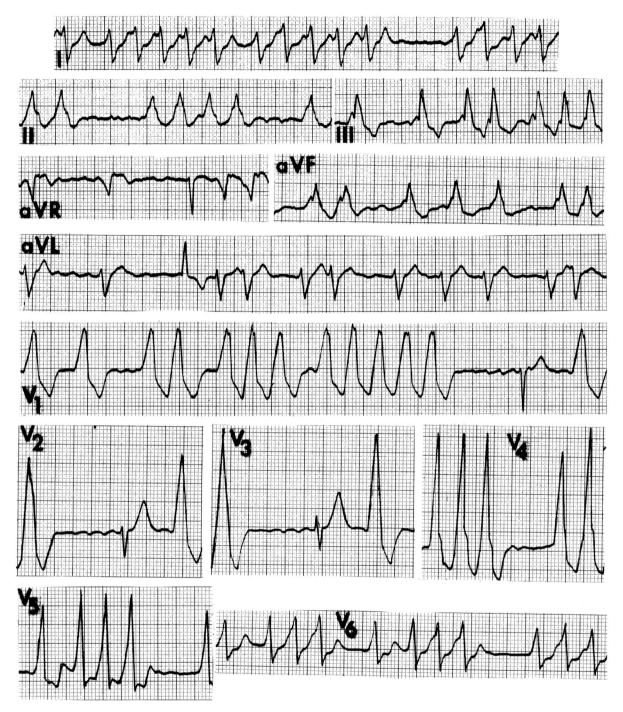

ECG III–72. *AF with Kent bundle conduction.* The cadence is grossly irregularly irregular. The QRS morphology is bizarre (rS in I, rR′ in aVF, R in V₁–V₅ with RS in V₆). The pauses represent failure of Kent bundle conduction. The narrow beats represent pure A–V nodal conduction.

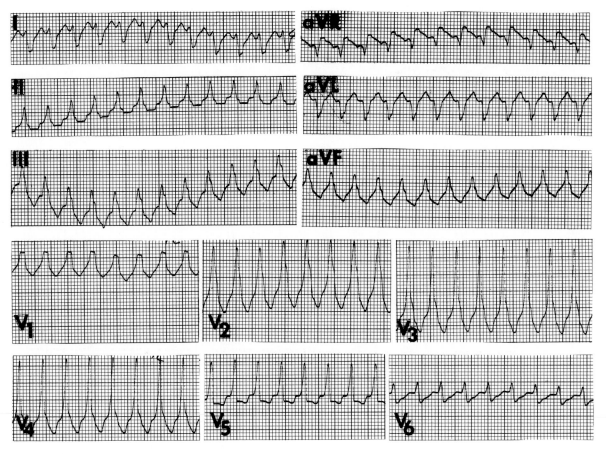

A

ECG III–73. *RSVT with antegrade Kent bundle conduction.* A. The rhythm is regular at 214 bpm. The QRS morphology is bizarre (rS in I, with R in II, III, and aVF,* R in V₁–V₅ and RS in V₆). The diagnosis would ordinarily be VT.

*RBBB with left posterior hemiblock would consist of a qR morphology in the inferior leads.

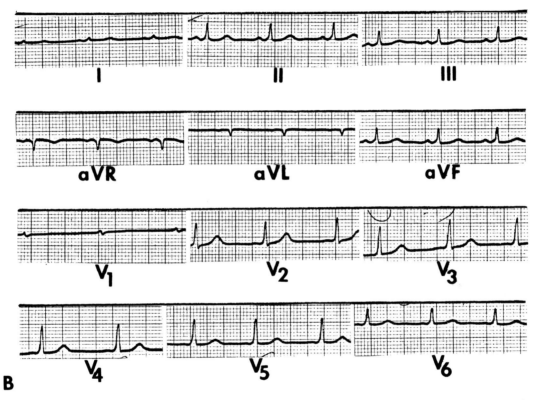

ECG III–73 (cont'd).   B. Examination of a previous ECG reveals small but definite delta waves in each lead. The polarity of the delta waves in each lead matches the polarity of the initial vectors of the beats during the tachycardia (III–73A), suggesting RSVT with antegrade Kent bundle conduction.

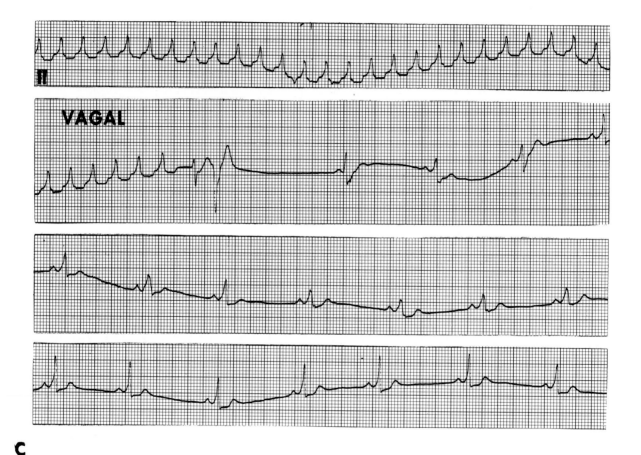

C

ECG III–73 (cont'd).   C. The rhythm breaks with vagal maneuvers (aramine drip). Note the delta waves in the sinus beats.

D

ECG III–73 (cont'd).   D. Twelve-lead ECG upon restoring sinus rhythm. Because of the lingering vagal influence on A–V nodal conduction, the delta waves are considerably more prominent than in III–73B.

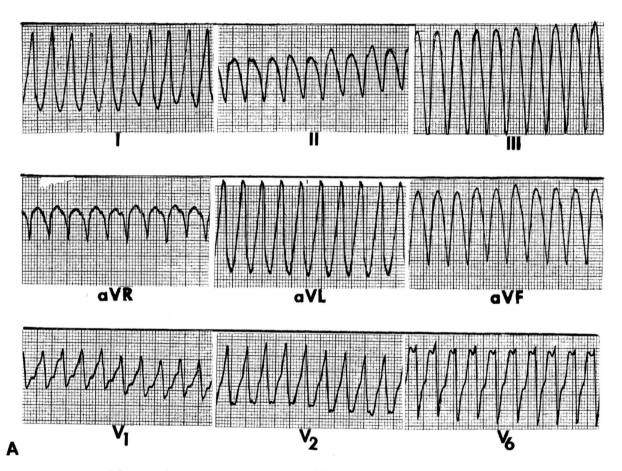

ECG III–74. *Atrial flutter with 1:1 conduction, RBBB and left anterior hemiblock.* A. There is a regular wide-QRS tachycardia at 230 bpm. The QRS morphology could be consistent with that of RBBB and left anterior hemiblock. VT is also a possibility in view of the rS in V_6.

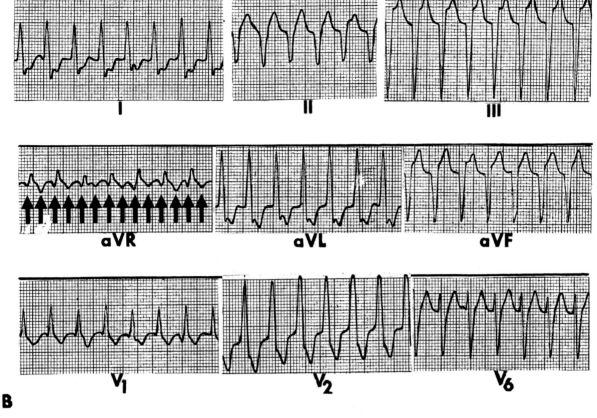

ECG III–74 (cont'd).   B. After digitalization, A–V conduction has decreased to 2:1. Flutter waves (arrows) are visible in Lead aVR. Patient has a history of atrial flutter, but had been taking quinidine without digitalis.

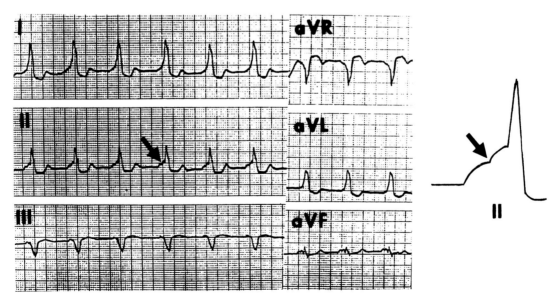

ECG III–75.   *W-P-W with marked delta waves.* The rhythm is sinus. The delta wave is so early it begins on the apex of the P-wave (arrow, Lead II). The wide, bizarre QRS-complexes indicate that A–V conduction is almost exclusively *via* the Kent bundle. The insert is an enlargement of Lead II.

Parasystole, Concealed Conduction, Intermittent Bundle Branch Block, Other Miscellaneous Arrhythmias, and Artificial Pacemakers

PARASYSTOLE

Under normal circumstances, the many latent pacemakers of the heart are continually penetrated and reset by the impulses arising in the S–A node. In this manner, they remain suppressed by the usually faster sinus. Occasionally, a latent pacemaker may temporarily acquire a protective shell of refractory tissue which prevents its penetration by the sinus (i.e., entrance block). The pacemaker may then reach threshold and discharge. Such a protected latent pacemaker is termed a *parasystole,* and may be located in the atria, junction, or ventricles. Upon firing, a parasystolic focus may find its impulse blocked either because the surrounding tissue has been rendered refractory by a sinus beat which it follows too closely, or because the immediately surrounding tissue is refractory due to intrinsic reasons (i.e., exit block).

On the ECG, a parasystole is recognized when a series of atrial, junctional, or ventricular extrasystoles are found to be related to each other, rather than either fixed-coupled to the dominant rhythm or randomly occurring. The interectopic intervals may be constant or varying. If varying, either the longer intervals are multiples of the shorter intervals, or all the intervals are multiples of some

shorter interval not present. In rare cases, the exit block around a parasystole may be of Wenckebach type. In cases of subjunctional or ventricular parasystole, fusion beats may be present, and must be counted when determining the interectopic intervals.

Occasionally, a parasystole may retrogradely conduct and reset the dominant pacemaker (e.g., a junctional or ventricular parasystole producing a retrograde-P-wave to reset the sinus; a ventricular parasystole retrogradely conducting to reset the junction [*via* manifest conduction which produces a retrograde-P-wave, or concealed conduction which does not]). In such cases, if the rate of the dominant pacemaker is less than double the rate of the parasystole, *the latter,* once it appears, *will continually reset the former.* This "reversed coupling" is manifested as sinus or junctional rhythm with fixed-coupled extrasystoles in bigeminy. That the extrasystoles represent a parasystole is detected only when one of them fails to retrogradely conduct and reset the dominant pacemaker, thus breaking the cadence. The subsequent extrasystole would retain the identical interectopic interval, but lose its fixed coupling to the previous dominant beat.

Unfortunately, the diagnosis of parasystole is

237

frequently not clear-cut. The intrinsic rate of a parasystole may slightly vary (because of local factors, changing autonomic tone, or "electrotonic" factors [influence by the rate of the dominant pacemaker]). It has also been shown that, despite entrance block, during a brief portion of the parasystolic cycle, the focus may be entered and reset. Thus, a critically timed beat may throw off one's interval measurements. What is important to remember is this: parasystole is a clinically benign rhythm. If one sees numerous, unifocal, non-fixed-coupled PVCs, and a number (but not all) of the intervals are suggestive of a parasystole (with the interval measurements appropriate to within, say, 200 msec.), one can simply say that a ventricular parasystole is likely.

CONCEALED CONDUCTION

Concealed conduction of an impulse cannot be seen directly, but *is inferred from its effect on the subsequent beat*, the latter being either reset or delayed or blocked in its conduction. Many manifestations of concealed conduction have already been encountered; the concealed retrograde penetration of the conducting system by a PVC, rendering it refractory to the subsequent sinus beat to produce a "full compensatory pause" is one common example. The beats initiating concealed conduction never reach their destination: sinus, atrial, and junctional beats do not antegradely reach the ventricles to produce a QRS; ventricular and junctional beats do not retrogradely reach the atria to produce a retrograde-P-wave. Yet, these impulses conduct far enough to reset a dominant pacemaker, or to render a portion of the conducting system fully or partially refractory to the next beat.

The various manifestations of concealed conduction are reviewed in Table IV–1. Several comments should be made.

During junctional rhythm, the junction is susceptible to being reset by (1) concealed antegrade conduction of a sinus-P or PAC (during periods of A–V dissociation), (2) concealed retrograde conduction of a PVC, or (3) concealed reentry (concealed ventricular echo arising from manifest or concealed retrograde conduction terminating a V–A Wenckebach period). When a PVC occurs during junctional rhythm it occasionally does not interrupt the junctional rhythm (i.e., little or no concealed retrograde conduction). More often, however, the junction is affected by the PVC. If concealed retrograde conduction reaches the level of the junctional pacemaker, the latter is reset. If it stops in the conducting system before reaching the pacemaker site, the next junctional impulse occurs

on time, but, owing to the refractoriness of the distal conducting system, is blocked or delayed. Stated in a somewhat different way, when one encounters a junctional rhythm with PVCs in bigeminy, one cannot ascertain the true junctional rate. It may equal (1) the apparent rate (no or little concealed conduction, junction is conducted with or without delay), (2) double the apparent rate (concealed penetration of the distal conducting system resulting in 2:1 H–V block), or, (3) between the apparent rate and double it (concealed retrograde conduction with reset of the junction) (review Figure I–4). Only when the PVC finally fails to occur or when there is a change in the degree of concealed conduction can the true junctional rate be determined.

JUNCTIONAL RATE CHANGES

The causes of a change of the junctional rate in junctional rhythm have been discussed in Section I (review pp. 17–18). Junctional arrhythmia is seen in young healthy individuals, while transient slowing or suppression of an otherwise constant rate is confined to those with serious heart disease.

P–R INTERVAL VARIATION

Two distinct sets of P–R intervals during sinus rhythm at a constant rate suggest dual A–V nodal pathway conduction. The two intervals may alternate, occur randomly, or switch from one to another after an extrasystole. When alternating, A–V Wenckebach conduction may develop in one of the sets. In contradistinction to dual pathway conduction, first-degree A–V block may develop in some individuals at faster rates. Finally, there is one reported case of wildly but phasically fluctuating P–R intervals in an individual with congenital absence of the right vagus; respiratory-phasic vagal changes were being applied only to the A–V node, rather than to the S–A and A–V nodes in balance, as normally occurs.

SINUS TACHYCARDIA WITH PACs AND A–V CONDUCTION DISTURBANCE

Because of the many P-waves, short P–P intervals, and varying P–R intervals, the rhythm is usually impossible to analyze by "eyeball." A step-by-step approach, analyzing the P-waves first, is mandatory and is illustrated in ECG IV–18.

INTERMITTENT BUNDLE BRANCH BLOCK

Bundle branch block (BBB) may be complete or incomplete. Complete right or left BBB involves a QRS of at least 0.12 sec.; in incomplete right or left BBB, or in the case of a hemiblock, the QRS is less

TABLE IV–1. Manifestations of Concealed Conduction.

Event	Extent of Conduction (Farthest Site Reached)	Consequence
A. Concealed antegrade conduction of a sinus-P or PAC (no QRS produced).	Junction or lower A–V node	Reset of junctional pacemaker. Reentry to produce atrial echo.
B. Concealed antegrade conduction of a PJC (no QRS produced) 1. With manifest retrograde conduction (retrograde-P produced).	Antegrade: local Retrograde: atria	Production of "isolated" retrograde-P (mimicking a PAC).
2. With concealed retrograde conduction (no retrograde-P produced).	Antegrade: local Retrograde: local	First- or second-degree (pseudo-Mobitz II) block of subsequent sinus beat.
C. Concealed retrograde conduction of a junctional or ventricular beat (no retrograde-P produced).	A–V node	Block or delay of a subsequent sinus beat.
	Junction or subjunction (by a ventricular beat)	Block, delay, or reset of a subsequent junctional beat (during junctional rhythm).
	High A–V node	Reentry to produce ventricular echo.
D. Concealed antegrade conduction during reentry initiated by delayed retrograde conduction of a junctional beat during junctional rhythm (no ventricular echo produced). 1. With manifest initial retrograde conduction (retrograde-P produced). 2. With concealed initial retrograde conduction (no retrograde-P produced).	Junction	Reset of junctional pacemaker (concealed ventricular echo).
E. Concealed retrograde conduction during reentry initiated by delayed manifest antegrade conduction of a sinus-P during SR with A–V Wenckebach period (no atrial echo produced).	High A–V node	Reentry to produce ventricular echo (ventricular echo from a concealed atrial echo) (review ECG II-35C).
F. Concealed antegrade conduction of AF or flutter (no QRS produced).	Proximal bundle branches	Abolition of favorable cycle-sequence comparison for functional aberration (review p. 161 and ECG III-44).
G. Concealed transseptal conduction and entry of distal bundle branch from the contralateral bundle branch during a supraventricular tachyarrhythmia with functional aberration.	Contralateral bundle branch	Sustained functional aberration (review Fig. III-4).
H. Concealed retrograde conduction of a ventricular (or ventricular-paced) beat in a patient with His bundle or unilateral/bilateral bundle branch block.	His-Purkinje system	Supernormal conduction of critically timed subsequent sinus beat.

than 0.12 sec. Complete block of a bundle branch means the ventricles are activated asynchronously, and may occur because of either (1) total failure of conduction in the bundle (3° block), or (2) severe delay of conduction in the bundle (1° block). In the latter case, should equal delay develop in the contralateral bundle branch, the ventricles are again activated synchronously, but only after considerable delay. An increased P–R interval followed by a narrow QRS thus results. Should even further slowing develop in the contralateral bundle, a further increased P–R interval followed by a wide QRS having the contralateral BBB pattern results.

In addition to incomplete and complete right and left BBB, Wenckebach conduction may rarely occur in the bundle branches (review ECG II–24). The development of a contralateral BBB pattern in a patient with complete right or left BBB, or of Wenckebach conduction in the contralateral bundle branch, or of the other hemiblock in a patient with complete RBBB plus a hemiblock all indicate severe bilateral bundle disease. As advanced infranodal block could occur at any time, the insertion of a pacemaker is indicated.

BBB may be fixed or intermittent. A classification of intermittent BBB is given in Table IV–2.

True intermittent BBB may be either random or rate-related, and may involve complete or incomplete right or left BBB, bifascicular block, a hemiblock, or left axis deviation with fixed LBBB. In random intermittent BBB, the block is seen at both fast and slow rates, and does not occur only after "long-short" cycle sequences. In some cases, the block occurs in a repetitive pattern (e.g., 2:1). Most rate-related BBB is tachycardia-dependent. The block appears at faster rates (above some critical rate), but not always following "long-short" sequences. In some cases, a "fatigue" effect is pres-

ent; that is, the block appears only after the rate has increased for a number of beats, and remains for a number of beats after the heart rate has decreased below the critical rate. Type I antiarrhythmic drugs, such as Quinidine, tend to accentuate "fatigue," whereas more marked increases in rate above the critical rate tend to reduce the effect. In some cases, as the rate increases, the QRS-complexes go through a transition of incomplete BBB before developing complete BBB. Bradycardia-dependent BBB is block which tends to occur only at slower heart rates. Much less common than the tachycardia-dependent variety, it is attributed to the decreased excitability of an injured bundle branch produced by a slow rise of the membrane potential during long cycles ("phase-4 depolarization").

What appears to be intermittent BBB may represent either no organic BBB, or fixed BBB with transient remission. Functional aberration can be induced in most individuals, and represents no organic BBB. It occurs only after suitable "long-short" cycle sequences, and, when sustained, continues only as long as the rapid rate continues. In many cases, it terminates before the heart rate slows. Transient remission of fixed BBB may occur for one of two reasons: (1) The antegrade conduction of an impulse may reach the affected bundle branch at the time of its supernormal phase (at the end of the T-wave of the previous beat). This occurs when a sinus beat closely follows a junctional, ventricular, or ventricular-paced beat, or when a PAC, PJC, or ventricular echo closely follows a sinus beat. In cases of supernormality, the last 0.04 to 0.08 sec. of the narrow beat's P–R interval coincides with the end of the T-wave of the previous beat. (2) Frequently, an early PAC is conducted with considerable first-degree A–V block, since it encounters a partially refractory A–V node. If the A–V nodal delay is marked, the QRS may itself be only minimally early. For such a beat, the interval between its depolarization of the affected bundle branch and that of the previous beat may, in fact, be slightly longer than the bundle branch interval between two sinus beats. In other words, great delay proximally, in the A–V node, may result in slight lengthening of the more distal H–H or bundle branch interval. This lengthening may exceed the critical interval needed for recovery of conduction in the affected bundle branch. Such a "gap phenomenon" is diagnosed when, in the presence of fixed BBB, a PAC with marked first-degree A–V block produces a narrow-QRS of only slight prematurity.

An early supraventricular beat terminating a

TABLE IV–2.   Intermittent Bundle Branch Block (BBB).

A. True intermittent BBB
  1. Random intermittent BBB
  2. Rate-related BBB
    a. Tachycardia-dependent (w/wo "fatigue")
    b. Bradycardia-dependent
B. Not true intermittent BBB
  1. Functional aberration/sustained functional aberration (no organic BBB)
  2. Fixed BBB with transient remission
    a. Supernormality
    b. "Gap phenomenon"
  3. Fixed BBB with QRS normalization (not true remission)
    a. Contralateral functional aberration with bilateral bundle slowing
    b. Fusion with an ipsilateral PVC

"long-short" interval may develop functional aberration. If there is fixed BBB resulting from severe slowing of conduction in the bundle, and the early beat develops similar contralateral functional slowing, the ventricles are activated synchronously, and a narrow-QRS results. QRS normalization *via* this mechanism is diagnosed when, in the presence of fixed BBB, an *early* supraventricular QRS (e.g., PAC, PJC, ventricular echo, or sinus beat) terminates a "long-short" sequence. That other beats with comparably short coupling intervals, but not terminating such "long-short" sequences, manifest BBB excludes bradycardia-dependent BBB. Considerable prematurity of the QRS effectively excludes the "gap" as a mechanism. Supernormality is excluded if the last 0.04 to 0.08 sec. before the early QRS occurs *after* the end of the T-wave of the previous beat. It must be remembered that the mechanism of functional slowing in the contralateral bundle does not represent actual transient remission of the patient's fixed BBB, let alone true intermittent BBB.

Finally, the fusion of a supraventricular beat showing a BBB with an ipsilateral PVC may result in a normalized QRS. To make this diagnosis, one must find a pure PVC which has a contralateral BBB pattern. The narrow, fusion beats are minimally early at most. Again, despite the normalized QRS, there is no real remission of the fixed BBB.

INTERMITTENT WOLFF-PARKINSON-WHITE (W-P-W) SYNDROME

Antegrade Kent bundle conduction (producing a delta wave) may be fixed or intermittent. Many Kent bundles do not conduct well antegradely at rapid heart rates. In other individuals, Kent bundle conduction may suddenly "drop out" at any heart rate. Kent bundle conduction may come and go sporadically or in some regular ratio (e.g., 2:1). When the heart rate is relatively rapid, the delta wave quite large, and Kent conduction 2:1, differentiation between 2:1 W-P-W and PVCs in bigeminy may be next to impossible. Vagal maneuvers, by slowing the heart rate and/or by decreasing A–V nodal conduction, may produce 1:1 Kent conduction, thus making the diagnosis. Occasionally, the delta wave is quite small and subtle. This may be particularly frustrating if, during the taking of the ECG, Kent conduction is completely "on" during the taking of some entire leads, and completely "off" during the others, thus excluding comparison of the beats within a given lead. In rare cases, delta waves are superimposed on beats already widened by left or right BBB (see ECG IV–25).

BIDIRECTIONAL TACHYCARDIA

This rhythm appears as a regular tachycardia with wide-QRS-complexes of alternating polarity in some of the leads. It most likely represents a markedly accelerated junctional rhythm with alternating BBB (or RBBB with alternating hemiblocks), and is seen most often in severe digitalis intoxication.

PACEMAKER ARRHYTHMIAS

Most pacemakers in use today are ventricular demand pacemakers. When the patient's heart rate drops below a pre-set interval, the pacemaker escapes and continues to fire at that rate until its pacing interval is preempted by another of the patient's own beats. (When a patient's own beat occurs, the pacemaker senses it and is suppressed.) Some models have a *rate hysteresis* feature; that is, the escape interval slightly exceeds the pacing interval.

Occasionally, a pacemaker apparently fails to sense the first portion of a widened QRS (PVC or supraventricular beat with BBB), yet senses all other beats normally. Such "late sensing" is not failure to sense, but a manifestation of the latency of the pacemaker (up to 0.16 sec.). It may take this time for the impulse to reach the tip of the pacemaker catheter, usually located at the apex of the right ventricle (see ECG IV–29). It is also not uncommon for a well-functioning pacemaker to completely not sense a sporadic PVC in the course of 24 hours; presumably, the intramyocardial activation pattern of the PVC is such that the net electrical potential at the site of the electrode is zero. Occasionally, the electrical potential of most of the patient's beats is too small to be normally sensed by the pacemaker. "Partial sensing" is the result. The pacemaker is reset, but by less than one complete sensing interval. The problem can be corrected by increasing the pacemaker's sensitivity or by repositioning the electrode to a more favorable site.

A drop in the pacemaker rate of 5 to 10 bpm usually indicates battery depletion and impending pacemaker failure. Out-and-out failure is manifested as any or all of the following: (1) failing to sense, (2) firing, but failing to capture, (3) failing to fire. All are present in ECG IV–30.

A pacemaker does not sense QRS-complexes occurring during its refractory period (up to 400 msec., depending on the model). This means that early PVCs (i.e., with extremely short coupling intervals) are not sensed.

Finally, pacemakers may be inhibited by the patient's own non-cardiac myopotentials, particularly those of the diaphragm. In such instances, the pacemaker fails to fire during coughing, deep breathing, or certain motions, despite a slow heart rate. When the magnet, which converts the unit to fixed-rate mode, is applied, the pacemaker fires normally, despite coughing, etc. Correction consists of decreasing the pacemaker's sensitivity.

The new A–V sequential pacemakers will not be discussed here. Needless to say, malfunction of these units may result in quite complex pacemaker arrhythmias.

SECTION IV
Electrocardiograms

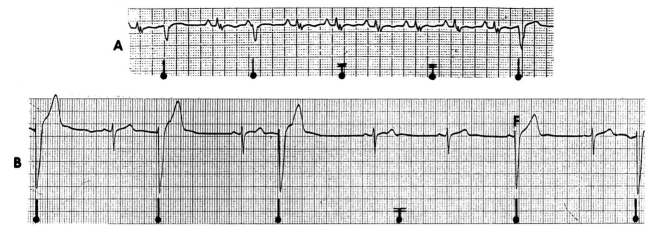

ECG IV–1. *Ventricular parasystole.* Unifocal non-fixed-coupled PVCs are present. A. The long PVC cycle is equal to three short cycles. B. One fusion beat (F) is present. The long PVC cycle is equal to two short cycles. (The basic parasystolic cycle length varies slightly.)

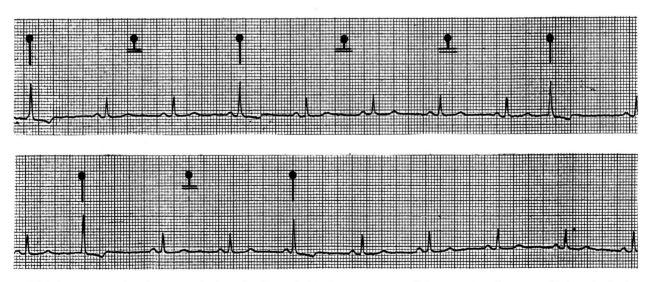

ECG IV–2. *Junctional parasystole.* Non-fixed-coupled PJCs are present. All junctional cycles are multiples of a basic cycle.

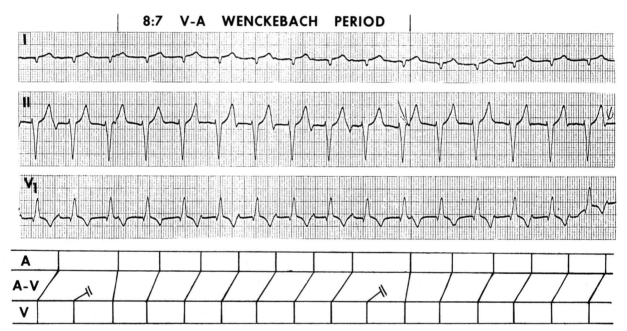

8:7   V-A   WENCKEBACH   PERIOD

ECG IV–3.   *Slow VT or rapid accelerated idioventricular rhythm with V–A Wenckebach periods.* The rate is 99 bpm. The QRS morphology is bizarre ("northwest" frontal plane axis and qR in V$_1$). Retrograde-P-waves follow the QRS-complexes by progressively increasing R–P intervals until a retrograde-P-wave fails to occur.

A = Atria; A–V = A–V Node; V = Ventricles.

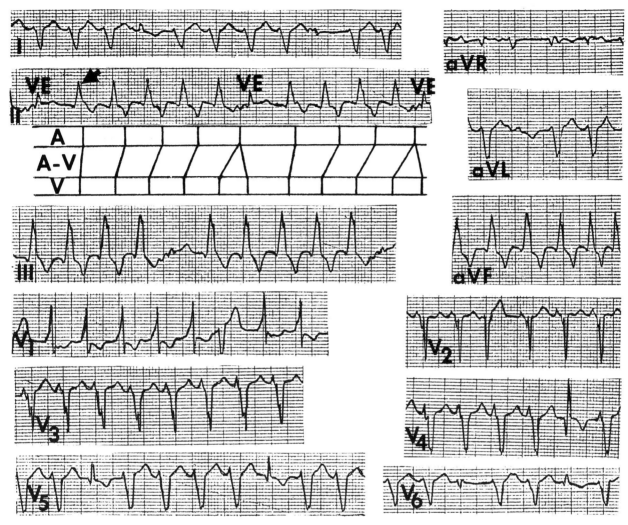

ECG IV–4. *VT with V–A Wenckebach periods culminating in ventricular echoes.* Bizarre, wide-QRS-complexes occurring at 135 bpm are periodically interrupted by narrow beats. By virtue of the QRS morphology and rate, as well as their not beginning with a "long-short" cycle sequence, these wide beats represent runs of VT. Turning to Lead II, the second, third, and fourth beats of the run beginning at the arrow are followed by deeper T-waves than the first beat. The first T-wave therefore represents the pure T-wave; the subsequent, deeper T-waves consist of pure T-waves plus superimposed retrograde-P-waves. The retrograde-P-wave following the fifth beat occurs later, at the end of the T. Following the narrow beat, the retrograde-P-wave is seen within the downstroke of the first wide-QRS-complex. The T-wave of the second wide-QRS is again deepened because of the increasing R–P interval. During the runs of VT there is therefore V–A conduction of Wenckebach type. The early, narrow beats thus represent ventricular echoes (VE); these terminate the A–V Wenckebach periods. Perusal of the ventricular echoes in all 12 leads reveals an acute inferolateral MI.

A = Atria; A–V = A–V Node; V = Ventricles.

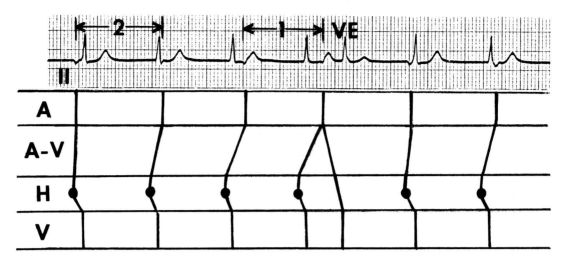

ECG IV–5.   *Accelerated junctional rhythm with V–A Wenckebach periods and a ventricular echo (VE).* The fact that the retrograde P–P cycle preceding the ventricular echo (1) is shorter than the first retrograde P–P cycle (2) indicates accelerated junctional rhythm with V–A Wenckebach conduction rather than A–V dissociation between accelerated junctional rhythm and an ectopic atrial pacemaker.

A = Atria; A–V = A–V Node; H = Bundle of His; V = Ventricles; VE = Ventricular Echo.

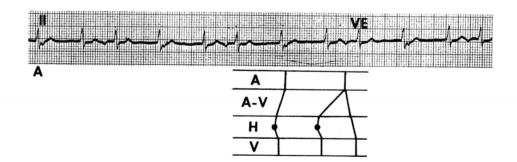

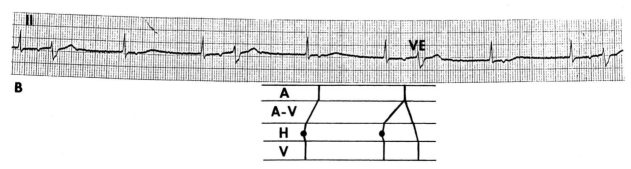

ECG IV–6.   *Junctional rhythm with V–A Wenckebach periods and ventricular echoes (VE) in trigeminy.* A. The junctional rate is accelerated at 83 bpm. B. The junctional rate is 45 bpm. The ventricular echoes manifest functional aberration.

A = Atria; A–V = A–V Node; H = Bundle of His; V = Ventricles.

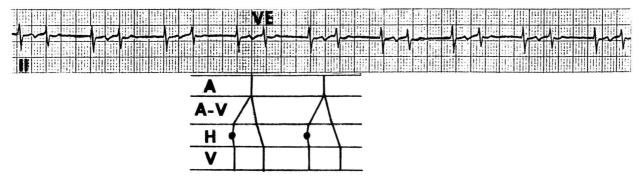

ECG IV–7. *Accelerated junctional rhythm (98 bpm) with ventricular echoes in bigeminy.* The ventricular echoes (VE) demonstrate mild functional aberration. The alternate explanation of this rhythm is ectopic atrial rhythm with accelerated junctional escapes in bigeminy. This is less likely, since one would expect an element of A–V block to accompany such junctional acceleration under the usual circumstances of digitalis toxicity; sinus or ectopic atrial P-waves arising in the Ts of the junctional beats would be unlikely to conduct, particularly with a P–R interval of only 0.16 sec. If the junction was accelerated due to catecholamine excess or cardiac surgery/trauma, one would ordinarily expect a faster atrial rate. Finally, confirmation of retrograde P-wave morphology in all 12 ECG leads would strongly support the proposed diagnosis. In either case, the junction is accelerated, A–V conduction is intact, and the sinus is relatively slow (60 bpm or less).

A = Atria; A–V = A–V Node; H = Bundle of His; V = Ventricles.

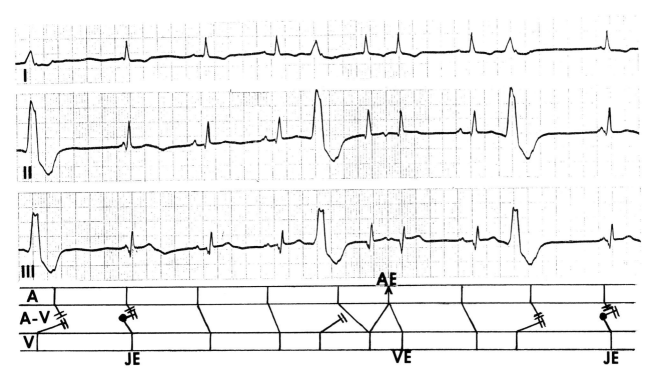

ECG IV–8. *First-degree A–V block resulting from concealed conduction of a PVC and leading to A–V nodal reentry.* The basic rhythm is sinus. Three PVCs are present. The first and third PVCs retrogradely penetrate the A–V node, rendering the node refractory to the next P-wave (in the T-wave of the PVC). The following P-wave would have conducted, but is pre-empted by a junctional escape (JE). The second PVC does not penetrate the A–V node as deeply. The following P-wave is able to conduct, but with significant first-degree A–V block.* Such critical antegrade conduction delay results in A–V nodal reentry, producing an atrial echo (AE) followed by a ventricular echo (VE).

A = Atria; A–V = A–V Node; V = Ventricles.

---

*The second PVC is therefore partially interpolated.

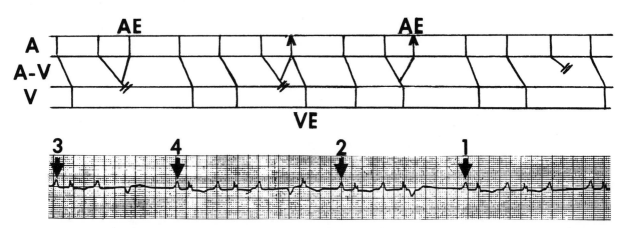

ECG IV–9. *Manifestations of concealed conduction during A–V Wenckebach periods.* Arrow #1 marks the beginning of a typical 3:2 A–V Wenckebach period. Arrow #2 marks the beginning of an A–V Wenckebach period which terminates in an atrial echo (AE). Arrow #3 begins another A–V Wenckebach period. In this sequence, the second P-wave fails to reach the ventricle, but penetrates the A–V node with sufficient delay and depth to produce an atrial echo. Finally, in the sequence beginning with arrow #4, the third P-wave again produces an atrial echo without having reached the ventricle. In this case, however, the atrial echo is followed by a ventricular echo (VE). Thus, in sequences 3 and 4, the atrial echo is a manifestation of concealed antegrade penetration of the A–V node by the preceding sinus-P-wave. (Reproduced by permission from Pick, A., and Langendorf, R.: Approaches to the diagnosis of complex A–V junctional mechanisms. *In* Mechanisms and Therapy of Cardiac Arrhythmias. Edited by L.S. Dreifus and W. Likoff. New York, Grune & Stratton, Inc., 1966.)

A = Atria; A–V = A–V Node; V = Ventricles.

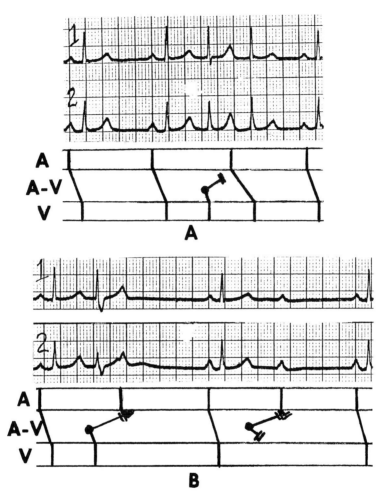

ECG IV–10. *Manifestations of concealed conduction produced by PJCs.* A. The basic rhythm is sinus. Concealed retrograde penetration of the A–V node by a PJC causes the subsequent sinus beat to be conducted with delay. B. The first PJC retrogradely penetrates farther into the A–V node, rendering it refractory to the next sinus beat. This PJC conducts antegradely with functional aberration of RBBB. Following the next sinus beat, there is a *second junctional discharge.* Because it terminates a more markedly "long-short" cycle sequence, this PJC encounters functional trifascicular block in its antegrade conduction, and is thus unable to produce a QRS. Like the first PJC, however, it retrogradely penetrates the A–V node, rendering it refractory to the subsequent sinus beat. Since this PJC is concealed, the impression of a sudden dropped beat is created ("pseudo-Mobitz II"; review ECG II–36).
A = Atria; A–V = A–V Node; V = Ventricles.

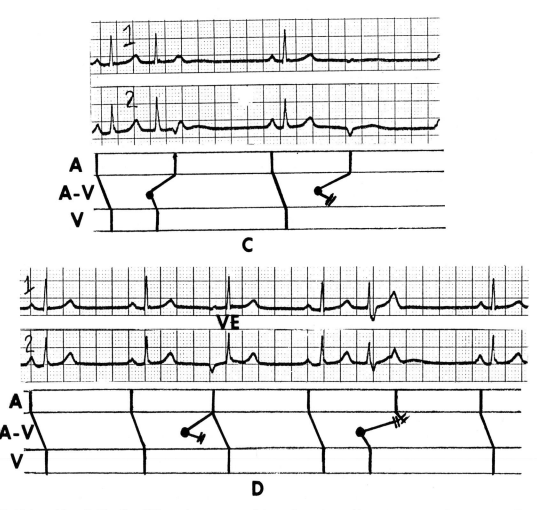

ECG IV–10 (cont'd).   C. The first PJC conducts retrogradely to the atria, producing a retrograde-P-wave. Following the subsequent sinus beat, a concealed PJC (i.e., no antegrade conduction due to functional trifascicular block) also conducts retrogradely to produce a retrograde-P. D. Following the first two sinus beats, a concealed PJC produces a retrograde-P-wave. In this case, the retrograde-P is followed by a ventricular echo (VE). Following the subsequent sinus beat, a second PJC is conducted with functional aberration of RBBB. The sinus-P-wave immediately following this PJC cannot conduct because of concealed penetration of the A–V node by the PJC. (Reproduced with permission from Childers, R.: Concealed conduction. Med. Clin. North Am., *60:*149, 1976.)

A = Atria; A–V = A–V Node; V = Ventricles.

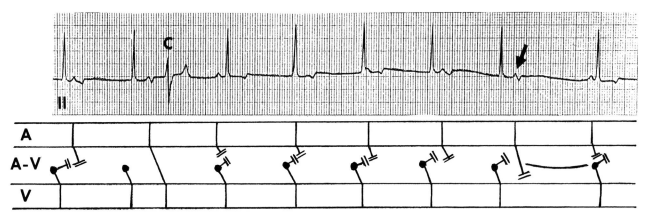

ECG IV–11. *Resetting of a junctional pacemaker by concealed antegrade conduction of a sinus-P-wave.* There is incomplete A–V dissociation between junctional rhythm at 55 bpm and the sinus at 49 to 52 bpm. There is one sinus capture (C) with functional aberration (RBBB + left anterior hemiblock). Following the capture, there is a period of A–V dissociation during which the P-waves move rightward into then out and away from the QRSs. One P-wave (arrow) penetrates the conducting system all the way to the level of the junctional pacemaker, thereby resetting it. However, the P-wave fails to reach the ventricle and make a QRS. The junction is thus reset by concealed antegrade conduction of a sinus-P-wave. (Reproduced with permission from Childers, R.: Concealed conduction. Med. Clin. North Am., *60:*149, 1976.)
   A = Atria; A–V = A–V Node; V = Ventricles.

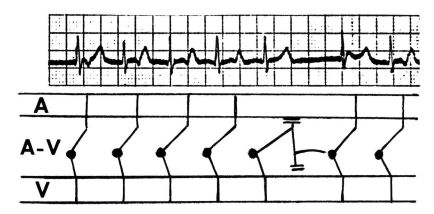

ECG IV–12. *Resetting of a junctional pacemaker by an abortive (concealed) ventricular echo.* The rhythm is an accelerated junctional rhythm at 110 bpm. The first four beats are followed by retrograde-P-waves; the R–P intervals progressively increase (i.e., V–A Wenckebach period). The fifth junctional beat fails to produce a retrograde-P-wave, but an unexplained pause follows the QRS. Although the atria were not reached, there was, in fact, concealed retrograde penetration to the highest reaches of the A–V node. From the upper A–V node, there was an attempt at antegrade reentry. The impulse reached the lower junction, beyond the region of the junctional pacemaker, but did not reach the ventricles. Thus, although a QRS was not made, the junction was reset by an abortive ventricular echo arising from concealed retrograde conduction. This ECG also illustrates that the atrium is not necessarily a part of the reentry circuit. (Reproduced with permission from Langendorf, R., and Pick, A.: Manifestations of concealed re-entry in the atrioventricular junction. Eur. J. Cardiol., *1/1:*11, 1973.)
   A = Atria; A–V = A–V Node; V = Ventricles.

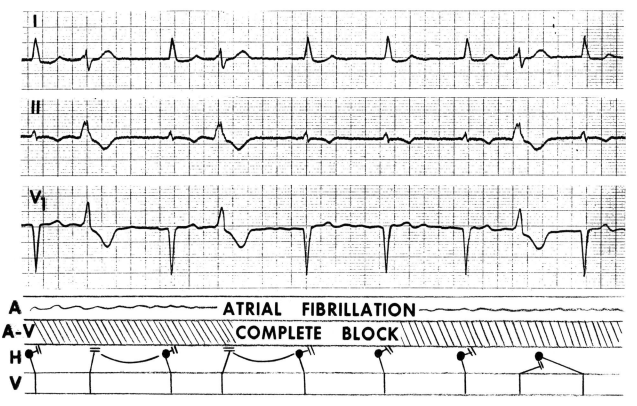

ECG IV–13.   *Effects of PVCs on junctional rhythm.* The basic rhythm is junctional at 55 bpm. There is underlying AF with complete block of the A–V node. The first two PVCs produce concealed retrograde penetration of the bundle of His. The junctional pacemaker is thus entered and reset. The third PVC's retrograde conduction does not reach the junctional pacemaker; however, the next junctional beat encounters a partially refractory distal conducting system, and is thus conducted with considerable delay.

A = Atria; A–V = A–V Node; H = Bundle of His; V = Ventricles.

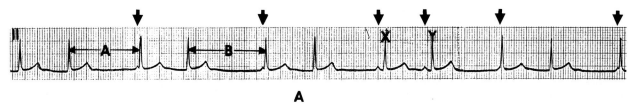

A

ECG IV–14.   *Junctional arrhythmia.* A. Coexisting sinus and junctional arrhythmia. There is marked sinus arrhythmia (arrows). X and Y are possible sinus captures. The rest of the QRSs are junctional (i.e., incomplete A–V dissociation). Although the QRS pattern appears to be bigeminal, the long and short cycles are, respectively, not precisely equal, thus excluding 3:2 H–V Wenckebach conduction (compare long cycles A and B). The QRS irregularity is therefore due to junctional arrhythmia, presumably because the pacemaker is located high in the junction, where it is subject to considerable vagal influence. This rhythm strip was obtained from an asymptomatic, young, healthy adult.

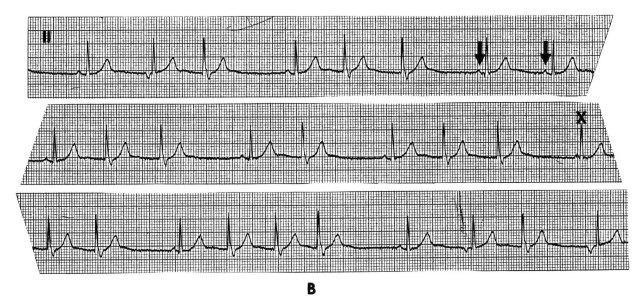

B

ECG IV–14 (cont'd).   B. The sinus rate is 57 bpm (arrows). Although there are a number of sinus captures, most of the QRSs are either preceded or followed by retrograde-P-waves. The rate of these junctional beats varies from less than 43 to 90 bpm. When the junction slows, the sinus emerges after being reset from the last retrograde-P. A–V dissociation occurs only at beat X. As in ECG IV–14A, the patient was an asymptomatic, young, healthy adult.

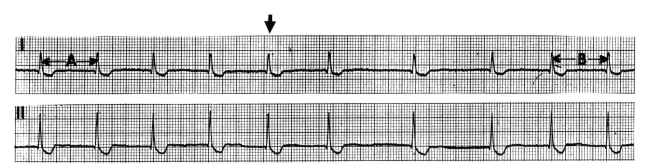

ECG IV–15.   *Spontaneous slowing of accelerated junctional rhythm.* There is an accelerated junctional rhythm at 72 bpm. The underlying rhythm is AF with complete A–V (nodal) block. At the arrow, the rhythm transiently slows. R–R intervals A and B are identical. Such slowing is rare, and is seen only in very sick hearts; in this case, the patient was digitalis-toxic. In such patients, slowing is more likely to occur following an extra, early beat (surpraventricular capture or an extrasystole) than as a spontaneous event.

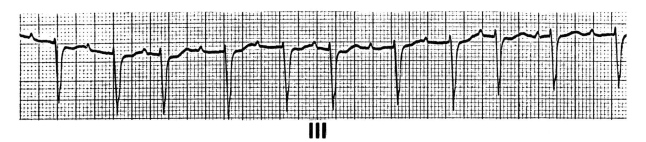

ECG IV–16.   *Dual A–V nodal pathway conduction.* The sinus rate is 100 bpm. There are 2 sets of P–R intervals (0.16 and 0.28 sec.).

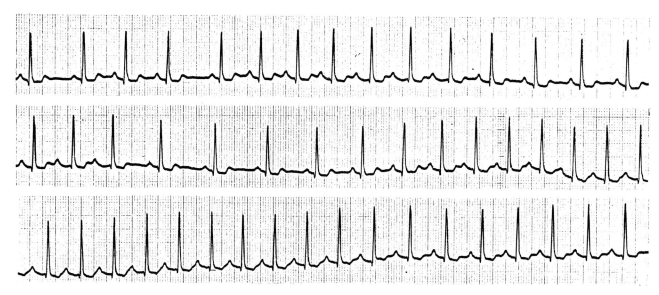

ECG IV–17. *Rate-related first-degree A–V block.* There is sinus arrhythmia. In contradistinction to ECG IV–16, the P–R intervals gradually increase as the rate increases, and gradually decrease as the rate decreases.

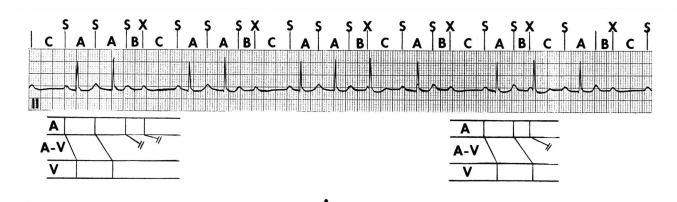

A

ECG IV–18. *Sinus tachycardia, A–V Wenckebach periods, and PACs.* A. First, mark each P-wave. Notice that there are three sets of P–P intervals. The P-waves terminating the "B" intervals are very early, and are clearly PACs (X). "A" is therefore the basic sinus rate (117 bpm). "C," which is slightly longer than "A," is the interval between the PAC and the returning sinus-P. Note that consecutive sinus-P-waves (S) conduct with increasing P–R intervals. The PACs, which are nonconducted, terminate these A–V Wenckebach periods, in some cases before, in other cases after a dropped beat has occurred.

A = Atria; A–V = A–V Node; V = Ventricles; S = Sinus-P; X = PAC.

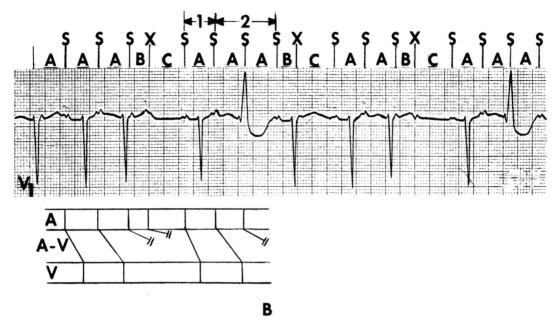

B

ECG IV–18 (cont'd). B. Analyze the rhythm strip like ECG IV–18A. Two of the QRSs are conducted with functional aberration of RBBB. (Note that the initial r-wave of the rSR' of these two beats is part of the QRS and *not* the initial deflection of a P-wave.) The sinus-P is completely buried within the widened QRS-complex. Since cycle 2 is exactly twice sinus cycle 1, cycle 2 must contain another sinus-P-wave. It times out to be completely within the QRS. The three PACs are nonconducted and terminate A–V Wenckebach sequences.

A = Atria; A–V = A–V Node; V = Ventricles; S = Sinus-P; X = PAC.

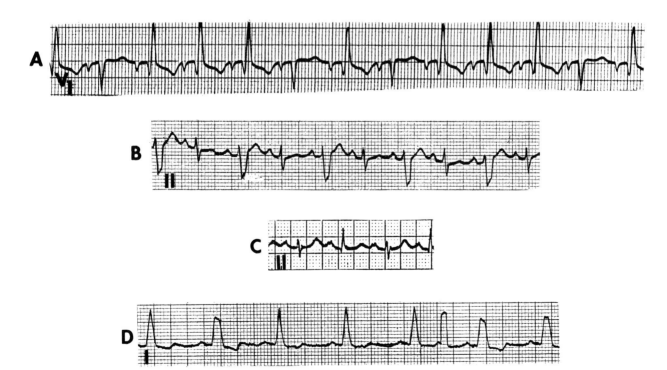

ECG IV–19. *Random intermittent bundle branch block.* A. Intermittent RBBB. B. Intermittent RBBB + left anterior hemiblock. C. Intermittent left anterior hemiblock. D. Intermittent LBBB.

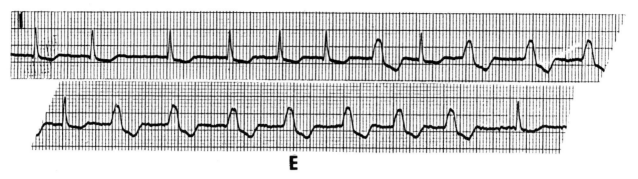

E

ECG IV–19 (cont'd).   E. Intermittent LBBB. The rhythm is AF. Note the LBBB does not appear only at faster rates or following a "long-short" cycle sequence.

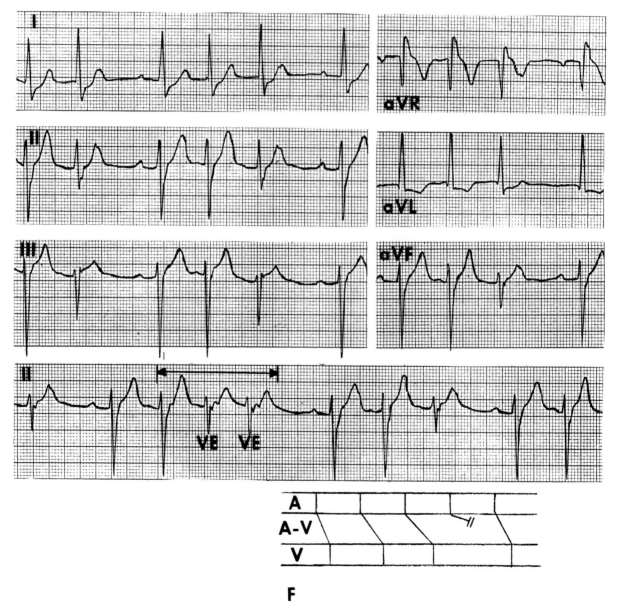

F

ECG IV–19 (cont'd).   F. RBBB with intermittent left anterior hemiblock. The rhythm is sinus tachycardia with A–V Wenckebach periods (note how the P-waves slightly deform the T-waves). One A–V Wenckebach period leads to several A–V nodal reentry loops (brackets).

A = Atria; A–V = A–V Node; V = Ventricles; VE = Ventricular Echo.

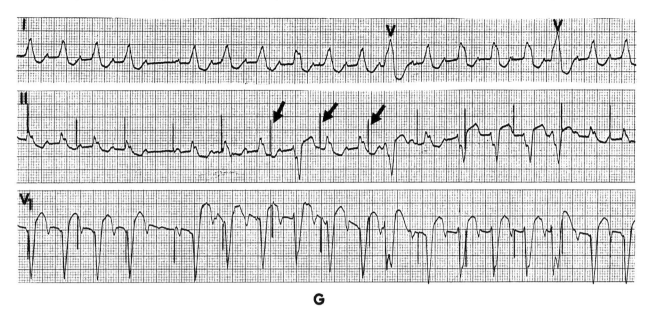

G

ECG IV–19 (cont'd). G. LBBB with intermittent left axis deviation. The rhythm is sinus tachycardia with one sudden dropped beat (Mobitz II 2° A–V block). Some of the beats have left axis deviation (rS in II) in addition to the LBBB. In addition, two PVCs (V) are present. These have LBBB-type morphology and preempt the P–R interval. Note the non-capturing pacemaker spikes (arrows). The patient, who had a history of advanced heart block, was admitted to the hospital following a syncopal episode; the malfunctioning pacemaker was replaced.

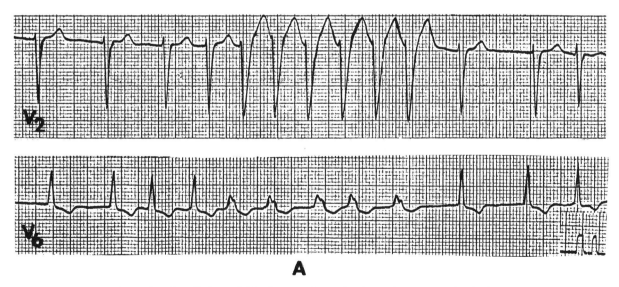

A

ECG IV–20. *Rate-dependent bundle branch block.* A. Tachycardia-dependent LBBB. The rhythm is AF. The runs of wide beats do not begin after particularly "long-short" cycle sequences. Although the rate is faster during the wide beats, the grossly irregular cadence in V₆ rules out VT.

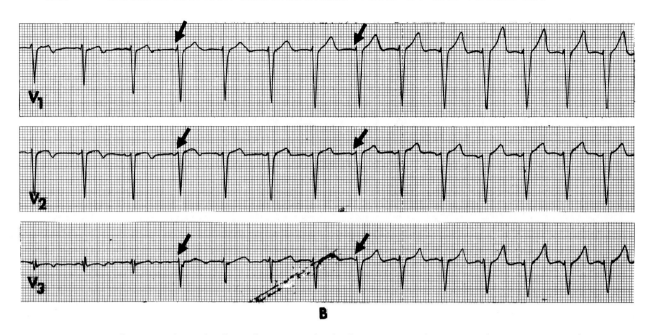

ECG IV–20 (cont'd).   B. Tachycardia-dependent LBBB. The rhythm is sinus. In this case, as the rate increases, the QRSs go through incomplete LBBB (first arrow) before developing complete LBBB (second arrow). C. Bradycardia-dependent bundle branch block. Review ECG II–43.

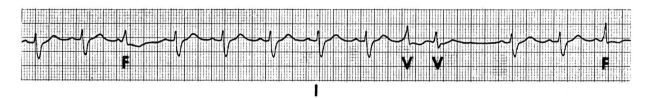

ECG IV–21.   *"Cancellation" of bundle branch block by fusion with an ipsilateral PVC.* The rhythm is sinus with RBBB. PVCs (V) arising from the right ventricle (i.e., LBBB-type morphology) are present. Two fusion beats (F) are present. These beats have narrow QRS-complexes, but shorter than normal P–R intervals.

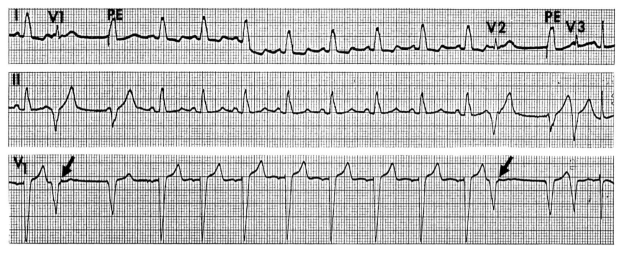

A

ECG IV–22. A. *Remission of bundle branch block during supernormal conduction.* The basic rhythm is sinus with LBBB and PVCs (V). The first two PVCs conduct retrogradely to the atria (arrows point to the retrograde-P-waves). The retrograde-P-waves reset the sinus, permitting an artificial ventricular pacemaker to escape (PE). Following the second pacemaker escape, there is another PVC (V3) which is not followed by a retrograde-P-wave. The sinus-P-wave immediately following the PVC is conducted with only a minimally prolonged P–R interval, and produces a narrow QRS. Presumably, the V3-PVC did not retrogradely penetrate the A–V node or even well into the bundle of His, since subsequent A–V conduction time is virtually normal. However, it did penetrate the bundle branches. The sinus-P-wave, occurring during the downstroke of the PVCs T-wave, reached the left bundle during its supernormal phase (at the end of the T-wave), and was able to conduct. The LBBB thus remitted for that one beat.

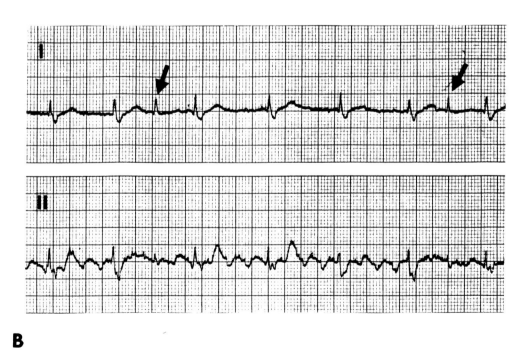

B

ECG IV–22 (cont'd). B. *Remission of bundle branch block in an early supraventricular beat.* The rhythm is AF with RBBB. Two early beats (arrows) show remission of the RBBB. The fact that each narrow beat is followed by another early beat manifesting RBBB indicates the remission is not attributable to bradycardia-dependent bundle branch block. The narrow beats come too early to be consistent with a "gap phenomenon" type of remission (see text). The remission must therefore be due either to supernormality (i.e., arrival of the atrial impulse at the right bundle at the time of its supernormal phase) or to functional aberration. In the latter case, the "long-short" cycle sequence results in functional delay in the left bundle equal to a pre-existent delay in the right bundle. Since the ventricles are activated synchronously, a narrow-QRS results. That the narrow beats are not merely ipsilateral PVCs in fusion is excluded by the absence of any pure PVCs (with LBBB morphology).

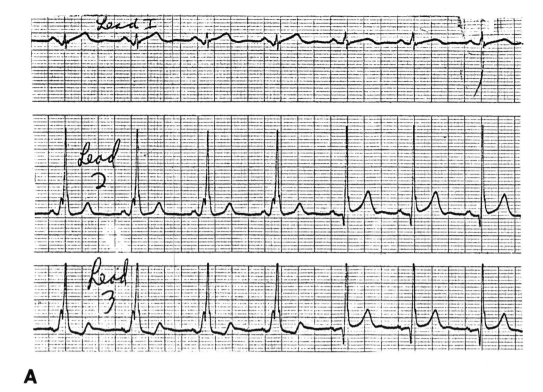

ECG IV–23.   A–C. *Intermittent delta wave in Wolff-Parkinson-White (W-P-W) syndrome.* The delta wave may be quite subtle (see C).

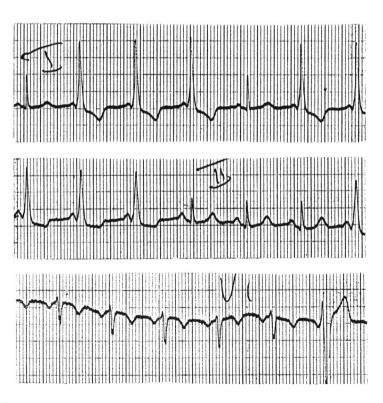

ECG IV–23 (cont'd).   B.

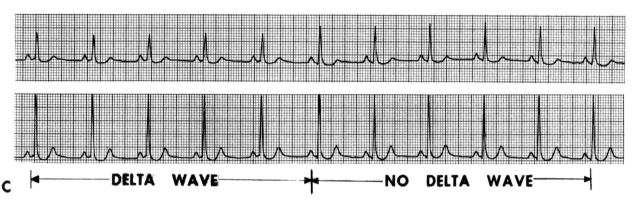

C |←————DELTA WAVE————→|←————NO DELTA WAVE————→|

ECG IV–23 (cont'd). C.

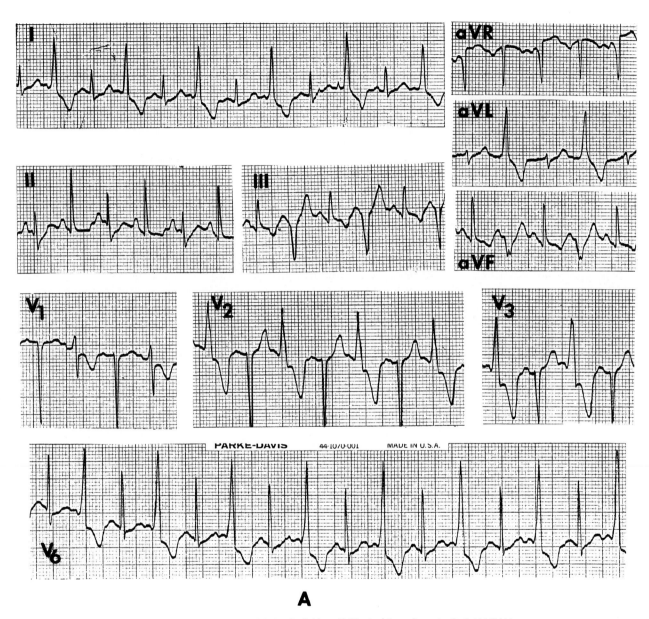

A

ECG IV–24.   *2:1 W-P-W mimicking PVCs in bigeminy. A. 2:1 W-P-W.*

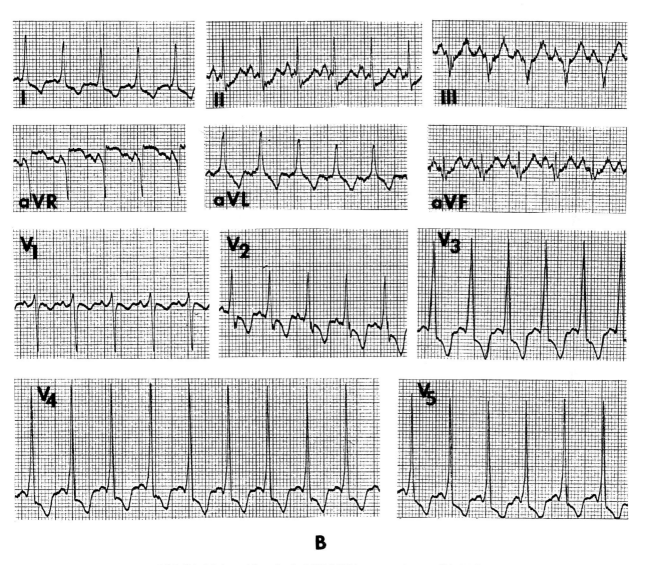

B

ECG IV–24 (cont'd).   B. 1:1 W-P-W (same patient as IV–24A).

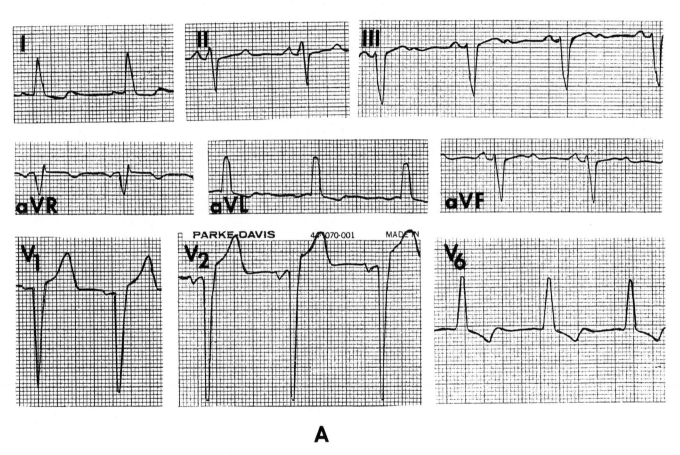

A

ECG IV–25. Intermittent W-P-W with baseline LBBB. (A–C same patient). A. LBBB.

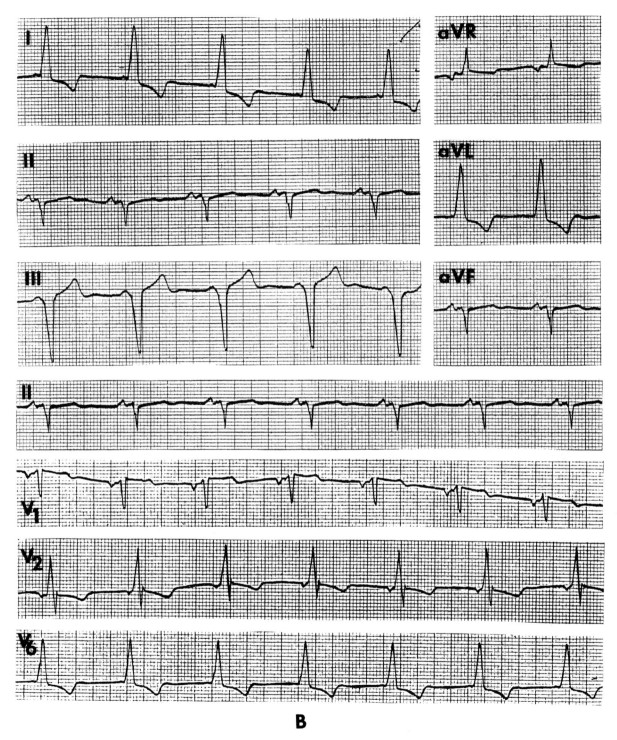

B

ECG IV–25 (cont'd). B. LBBB with W-P-W.

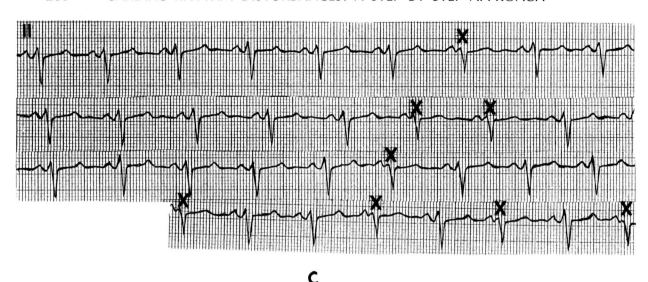

C

ECG IV–25 (cont'd). *C. LBBB with intermittent W-P-W.* The beats having a delta wave are indicated by "X."

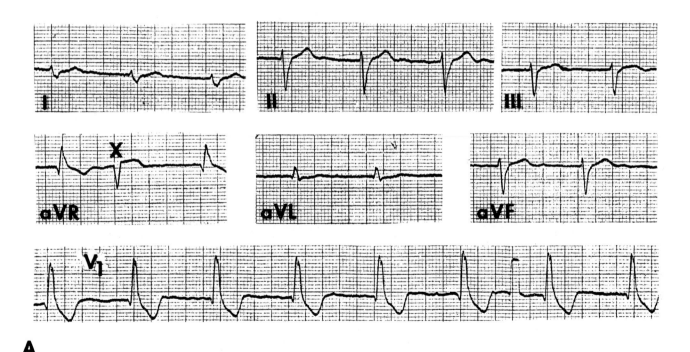

A

ECG IV–26. *Remission of digitalis intoxication in AF; deceleration of a subjunctional pacemaker.* A. The basic rhythm is AF with complete A–V (nodal) block. There is a regular rhythm with the QRS morphology of RBBB plus left anterior hemiblock. Because the previous ECG showed normal QRS-complexes and because the one conducted (i.e., early) beat (X) in this ECG has a narrow QRS, the rhythm presumably arises in the posterior fascicle of the left bundle branch. The subjunctional rate is accelerated at 62 bpm.

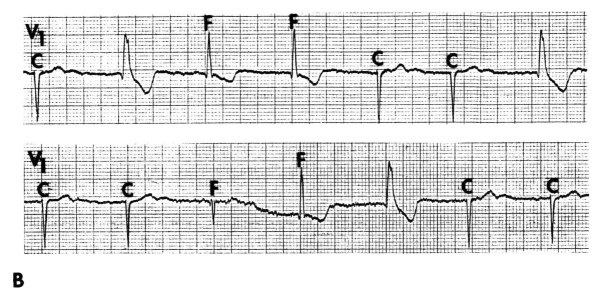

B

ECG IV–26 (cont'd).   B. Two days later. A–V conduction has greatly improved; numerous captures (C) are present. The subjunctional rate has slightly decreased to 60 bpm. Several fusion beats (F) are present.

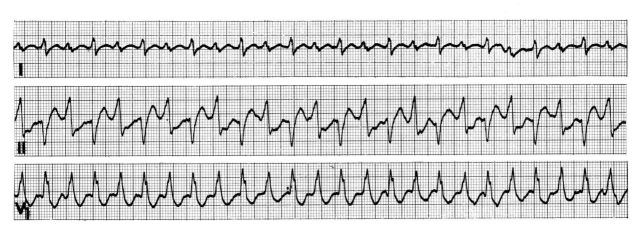

ECG IV–27. *Bidirectional tachycardia.* The rate is 167 bpm.

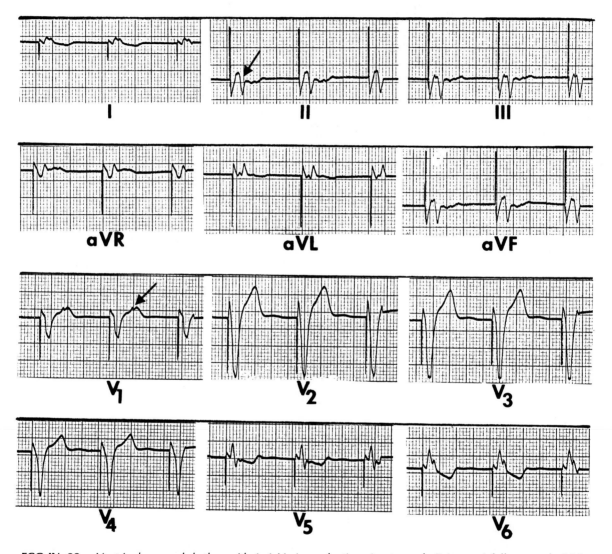

ECG IV–28. *Ventricular-paced rhythm with 1:1 V–A conduction.* A retrograde-P (arrows) follows each QRS.

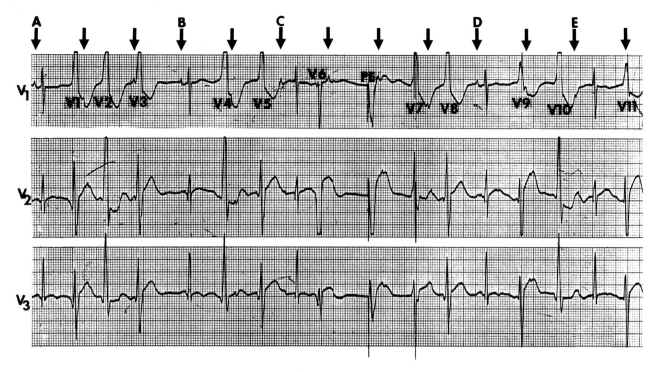

ECG IV–29. *Sinus rhythm with PVCs and pacemaker escapes.* The basic rhythm is sinus; first identify the P-waves (arrows). Five of the P-waves (A–E) are followed by sinus captures. PVCs (V) are present. P-waves C and E capture with long P–R intervals because of concealed retrograde conduction into the A–V node by the preceding PVC. Note that the initial portion of PVC-V6 is nearly isoelectric in Lead V_1, and could easily have been mistaken for a supraventricular beat if only V_1 had been examined. The nonconducted P-waves are situated relative to the PVCs so as to be unable to conduct. PVC-V6 is followed by an artificial ventricular pacemaker escape (PE). The pacemaker again fires in the middle of PVC-V7. The pacemaker is functioning normally. It "failed to sense" the first 0.08 sec. of the PVC because of normal latency of activation. The pacemaker is located in the right ventricle (note the LBBB-type of QRS it makes). The V7-PVC arises in the left ventricle (RBBB-type of QRS). The left ventricle is activated for at least 0.08 sec. before the PVC impulse reaches the pacemaker site in the right ventricle. Such latency may be as much as 0.16 sec.

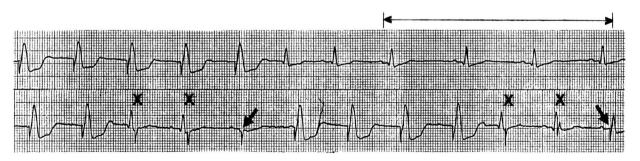

ECG IV–30. *Malfunctioning ventricular pacemaker.* The pacemaker fails to sense (X), for a time fails to fire (brackets), and, in one instance (first arrow), fires but fails to capture. (At the second arrow, the pacemaker is preempted by the simultaneously occurring sinus-QRS.)

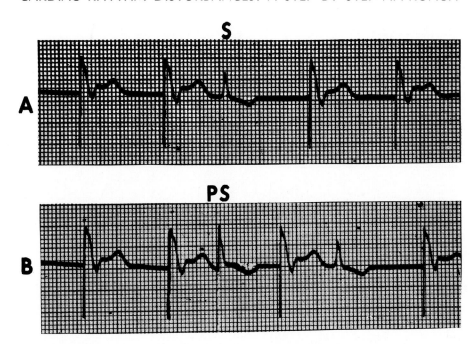

ECG IV–31.   *Partial sensing by a ventricular pacemaker.* A. The patient's own beat is properly sensed (S). B. The first of the patient's own beats is partially sensed (PS); that is, it is sensed, but the pacemaker is reset by less than one full cycle. The second beat is fully sensed. (From Costellanos, A., and Lemberg, L.: Pacemaker arrhythmias and electrocardiographic recognition of pacemakers. Circulation, *47*:1382, 1973. By permission of the American Heart Association, Inc.)

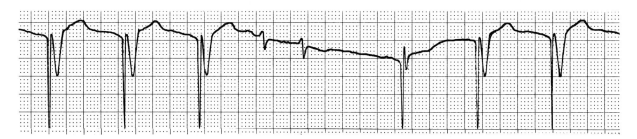

ECG IV–32.   *Rate hysteresis.* The initial pacemaker escape interval is longer than the pacing interval.

DEEP BREATHING

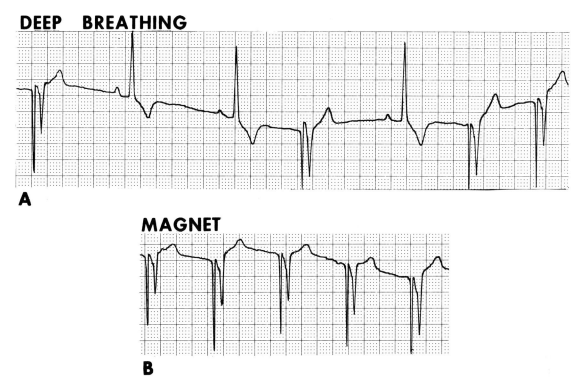

ECG IV–33. *Inhibition of a ventricular pacemaker by myopotentials.* A. During deep breathing, the pacemaker periodically fails to fire, permitting the slower sinus to escape. B. With the application of the magnet, the pacemaker is converted to fixed-rate mode, and fires appropriately. This problem was corrected by programming down the sensing sensitivity of the pacemaker.

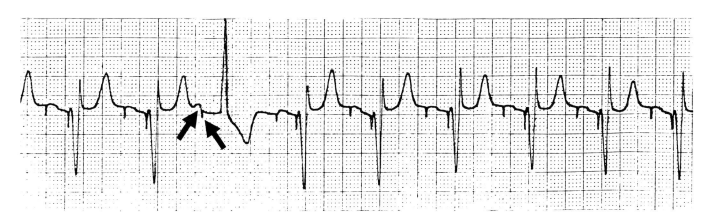

ECG IV–34. *A–V sequential pacemaker (DVI).* The atria and ventricles are paced. Both the atrial and ventricular pacing systems are QRS-inhibited. Although the patient's own P-wave has occurred (first arrow), the atrial pacemaker fires (second arrow) since it senses from the preceding paced QRS. The ventricular pacer is then preempted by the patient's own QRS (sinus capture). Following the sinus capture, the atrial pacemaker escapes, producing a paced P-wave. Approximately 0.22 sec. later, the ventricular pacemaker fires, producing a paced QRS. The paced "P–R interval" of 0.22 sec. is created because the ventricular pacing interval is 0.22 sec. longer than the atrial pacing interval. The ventricular pacemaker does *not* in any way interact with the atrial pacemaker.

INDEX

Page numbers in *italics* indicate figures and electrocardiograms; page numbers followed by t refer to tables.